TABIYAT

To
Vera, for her love and care,
and for the happiness we share

TABIYAT
Medicine and Healing in India
and Other Essays

FAROKH ERACH UDWADIA

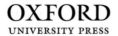
OXFORD
UNIVERSITY PRESS

OXFORD
UNIVERSITY PRESS

Oxford University Press is a department of the University of Oxford.
It furthers the University's objective of excellence in research, scholarship,
and education by publishing worldwide. Oxford is a registered trademark of
Oxford University Press in the UK and in certain other countries.

Published in India by
Oxford University Press
2/11 Ground Floor, Ansari Road, Daryaganj, New Delhi 110 002, India

First Edition published in 2018
Second impression 2018

ISBN-13 (print edition): 978-0-19-948015-9
ISBN-10 (print edition): 0-19-948015-X

ISBN-13 (eBook): 978-0-19-909161-4
ISBN-10 (eBook): 0-19-909161-7

Typeset in Sabon LT Std 11/14
by The Graphics Solution, New Delhi 110 092
Printed in India by Replika Press Pvt. Ltd

Contents

Preface   vii

1. A Knowledge of the Humanities and History
   Makes a Better Physician   1

2. The Fight against Infection: The Microbe Hunters   18

3. Medical Ethics   44

4. War and Medicine   74

5. Tabiyat: Medicine and Healing in India   100

6. The Lady with the Lamp   123

7. Music, the Mind and Medicine   142

8. Medicine in the Renaissance Era   172

9. Death   190

About the Author   209

Preface

My earlier book, *The Forgotten Art of Healing and Other Essays* (2009), has been a great success. I have succumbed to the request of many friends and patients to write another volume consisting of nine further essays on subjects related to medicine but divorced from its scientific and technical aspects.

The title that I have chosen for this book is *Tabiyat: Medicine and Healing in India and Other Essays*. The same heading is also the subject of the fifth essay in this volume. This essay is an edited version of a recorded extempore talk given by me at the Prince of Wales Museum (renamed Chhatrapati Shivaji Maharaj Vastu Sangrahalaya), on the occasion of the public viewing of exhibits related to the subject; the exhibits were brought to Mumbai from the Wellcome Collection through the kindness of the Wellcome Trust.

Among the many prevailing medical systems Indians use to preserve health and combat disease, Ayurveda remains the most important traditional system of medicine in this country. It is not sufficiently realized that from an overall perspective, many people in this country rely on Ayurveda and on other traditional medical systems rather than on Western medicine.

This essay traces the roots of Ayurveda, its philosophy, its rise and its achievements. It also discusses reasons for its stagnation after the eighteenth century in contrast to the rise of Western medicine from this period on. The essay mentions other systems of medicine prevailing in the country, with an added stress on folk medicine, which almost certainly must have preceded all other systems of medicine both in the East and West. It further goes on to compare Ayurveda to the Western system of medicine and submits that though Ayurveda even today remains a useful science and art in India, it cannot combat the numerous life-threatening illnesses that afflict Man.

'The Fight against Infection: The Microbe Hunters' describes the work of four great heroes in medicine. Three of these great men revolutionized the science of microbiology and infectious diseases and the fourth revolutionized the practice of surgery. It is of interest that these discoveries were made by observation, experimentation, intuition and by single-minded dedication. Interestingly, double blind randomized trials and evidence-based medicine, the 'mantras' of modern-day clinical medicine, were non-existent in that era of great discoveries.

The essay on 'Medical Ethics' was rather difficult to write, but I felt it imperative to do so, as there is indeed a sharp fall in the standard of medical ethics in our country. It is disheartening that the mutual trusting relationship between the physician and the patient—the doctor–patient bond, which lies at the heart of medicine—as also the bond between the medical profession and society stand eroded.

'War and Medicine' deals with a fascinating subject. The unmitigated horrors of war, the horrific mutilation of human bodies, and the destruction, famine, pestilence and death that war entails are best illustrated by the First and Second World

Wars. Yet, war has brought in its trail medical innovation and discoveries not only in the treatment of wounds and injuries but in many other branches of medicine and surgery. What amazes me is that out of this cauldron of death, destruction and disaster, some good can and did accrue.

'A Knowledge of the Humanities and History Makes a Better Physician' is the first of the nine essays in this book. It is based on an oration delivered to the public and the medical profession at the behest of the Research Society of the Sir Ganga Ram Hospital, Delhi. The recorded talk, with minor editorial corrections, forms the content of this work. It is unfortunate that very few in the medical profession have a reasonable acquaintance with the humanities and history. A study of the humanities, in my opinion, improves clinical judgement, allows a deep insight into the understanding of human nature, and breeds compassion and care. It allows a more holistic study of Man and their manifold responses to disease, and enables the physician to realize that medicine is in equal measure both an art and a science.

'The Lady with the Lamp' is the story of Florence Nightingale and the story of nursing as it exists today. It is the story of a young girl who dreamt to serve mankind by nursing the sick. It is a saga of courage, devotion and care, a magnificent obsession that was ultimately realized.

I have a passion for music and have truly enjoyed writing on this subject in the essay 'Music, the Mind and Medicine'. Music perhaps is the greatest of all art forms, even superior to literature and the visual arts. Music is related to every one of the many other art forms, in that like all other art forms, it has an aesthetic beauty. Yet, it is also unrelated in that it cannot be seen, is comprehended but cannot be translated, and bears no relation to the external world. I have given in this essay some thoughts on the origin of music, the mystery of music, the effects of music on the mind, music's inherent power and its relation to medicine. Finally, I end this essay with a philosophical discussion on the significance of music in our world.

'Medicine in the Renaissance Era' reflects on how the Renaissance was one of the great eras of human civilization that followed upon a period in history often termed the Dark Ages. It was as if humans, after groping through dark alleyways for several centuries, had at last opened the door to a beautiful sunlit garden. The Renaissance, chiefly known for its great contribution to art and culture, also produced great rebels who liberated medicine that had been fossilized by galenic beliefs for over a thousand years.

Last but not the least, we come to the essay on 'Death', the culmination of this work. Death is the only certainty in life, but is death the final irrevocable end or does it mark the beginning of a new life? We will never know, as no man or woman who has died has ever returned to tell the tale. The essay is a mixture of conjecture, philosophy and poetry. Let readers form their own opinions on this subject.

I have read and consulted many books and a number of references while writing these essays. They are too many to acknowledge singly but I need to especially acknowledge the book *War and Medicine* from the Wellcome Collection (2015). I have also used many cross-references in several chapters of this book. Among other books that were of great help were *Music and the Brain: Studies in the Neurology of Music* by Macdonald Critchley and R. A. Henson (1977), *Music and the Mind* by Anthony Storr (1992), *Musicophilia: Tales of Music and the Brain* by Oliver Sacks (2007), *Music Quickens Time* by Daniel Barenboim (2009) and *The Joy of Music* by Leonard Bernstein (1959). I have also consulted my own book *Man and Medicine—A History* (2000), as and when necessary.

The references I need to specially acknowledge are 'Deadly Comrades: War and Infectious Diseases' by M. A. Connolly and D. L. Heymann (2002) published in *The Lancet*; 'Is war good for medicine?' by Christopher Connell (2007) published in *Stanford Medicine Magazine*; 'The Neurochemistry of Music' by Mona Lisa Chanda and Daniel J. Levitin (2013) published in *Trends in Cognitive Sciences*; and 'Mozart, Music and Medicine' by E. K. Pauwels, D. Volterrani, G. Mariani and M. Kostkiewics (2014) published in *Medical Principles and Practice*. There are a number of poets, authors and quotations that I have consulted when writing on 'Death'. It is not possible to thank them individually but I acknowledge with gratitude the help they provided.

I owe a debt of gratitude to my wife, Vera Udwadia, for her patience and forbearance during the preparation of this work and for her reading and correcting the manuscript several times over. My very sincere thanks to Dr Khyati Shah, my research assistant, who has been associated with this work from its very inception. Her diligence and devotion were largely responsible for the completion of this book. I must also express my gratitude to my dear friend and distinguished surgeon, Dr Hirji S. Adenwalla. He has not only read the manuscript but offered excellent suggestions, many of which I have incorporated. My thanks to Neeraj Chavan for helping in the typing of the manuscript. I wish to acknowledge and thank the Wellcome Trust for the permission to print the pictures that illustrate the book. Finally I thank OUP for their unstinted help and co-operation in publishing this work.

1

A Knowledge of the Humanities and History Makes a Better Physician*

I believe that a knowledge of the humanities and history makes a better physician; it is a concept that is close to my heart. I passionately believe so. I am aware that I am addressing a scientific body but must at the outset warn you that the content of this essay is slightly loaded against science.

There is no greater saga in the history of mankind than the epic of medicine. Medicine emerged out of the mists of magical and empirical beliefs of the ancient civilizations. The trail of medicine has witnessed several twists and turns, victories and defeats, scintillating light and sombre darkness. Over five thousand years of history, medicine has evolved into

* This essay is based on an oration given by the author on the occasion of the opening of the Research Society of Sir Ganga Ram Hospital in Delhi.

a powerful force, an art, a science, a profession that has taken a quantum leap into the twenty-first century.

The first part of this essay is a brief discussion on the importance of the awareness of the history of medicine towards making a better physician. The history of medicine is important for several reasons. For one, it takes the physician back to his roots. Modern medical research and the evidence of palaeontology and anthropology affirm that medicine originated in magic and flourished as a priestly art. The roots of medicine lie in magic. Evil spirits entered the body through orifices and caused disease. The shamans of prehistoric and early historic civilizations exorcised these spirits. Then came the priest physicians of ancient Egypt and Sumer, who mixed magic and religion as twins of their priestly art and craft. The next step was empiricism, so that magic, religion and empiricism flourished together and constituted the practice of medicine. Empiricism is still very much a part of modern medicine, and magico-religious medicine can still be observed in a number of hidden corners of the world.

I do not propose to discuss the further evolution of medicine and the increasing role of science up to the present era. I would, however, like to emphasize that the panorama of medicine through the millennia is not just a chronological sequence of events and discoveries. Romance of medicine lies in the dynamic cavalcade of men and women who walked its trail. It is embedded in the heroes and the imposters, the caring and uncaring, who shaped its path. Also, medicine is not just about treating different diseased organ-systems. It embraces a more holistic concept of caring for man as a whole and treating each man or woman as a unique entity. A physician familiar with the history of medicine is better equipped to do so. He adds wisdom to knowledge, art to science, and humility to his prowess. An awareness of medical history also helps to build character. Lives of distinguished physicians and surgeons of the past, their discoveries, achievements and humanity are a source of inspiration and help to inculcate a modesty of being, which is the hallmark of great men and women. Finally, it is just as important to be aware of the mistakes and follies marking the path of medicine, as it is to know the strides that have led to its true progress. This inculcates within the physician an ability to question what he is taught or what he reads and encourages a spirit of enquiry that may well be translated into discoveries that push forward the frontiers of medicine.

The lessons of medical history are many, but I shall elaborate on just a few. The first and foremost is that there are limits to medicine. Every age since the beginning of history felt that it knew almost all that there was to be known, and every age was mistaken. In fact, the frustrations expressed towards medicine today are because expectations of people from medicine have always been more than what medicine can meet. The other important lesson of history is that truth is relative and never absolute. Many concepts and beliefs considered to be sanctified truths were proved to be false at another time and age. Unquestionably, many aspects of contemporary medicine about which so many are so proud may prove only relatively true or false, or even harmful another fifty to hundred years from now. Awareness of this fact in medical history teaches humility, tolerance and a respect for views which differ from current teaching. It counters the hubris of both science and of the physician who is exclusively immersed and steeped in the science of today.

Medicine can be considered as an edifice, broad-based and reaching upwards into the skies. Every age and culture has contributed a worthy stone or brick towards this edifice. The lesson we learn from medical history is that but for the foundations laid by our great predecessors, this edifice of medicine would not be there, so that contemporary medicine would perhaps have been different and not so successful.

The history of medicine like the history of mankind is a chronicle of change. Had it not been so, both civilization and medicine would have been fossilized centuries or millennia earlier. The lesson we can predict is that the shape of medicine years from now may be unrecognizable from what it is today.

Finally, perhaps the most important lesson in the history of medicine is that the soul and substance of medicine lies in its humanism and its humanity. Humanity is the sensibility that enables a physician to feel for the distress and suffering of a patient prompting him to give relief.

Let us now very briefly remember just a few of the great predecessors who illuminated the trail of medicine. In ancient Egypt, magic, religion and empirical medicine existed side by side. The Ebers papyrus and the Edwin Smith papyrus illustrate the scope of medicine and surgery five thousand years ago. I would like to present at this stage an individual, a character, who epitomizes and illustrates the very core and substance of today's discourse. From the mists of antiquity about 2,700 years before the birth of Christ, there emerged for the first time in recorded history the vivid personality of a great physician. His name was Imhotep (meaning, 'he who comes in peace'). One could not even today find a more multifaceted personality. He was vizier to the Pharaoh Zoser, and also his architect and high priest. He was renowned as a sage, philosopher, scribe, artist and astronomer. He built the first step pyramid at Sakkhara, the oldest extant stone structure in the world. He introduced bas-reliefs and the fluted shaft, symbolizing Egyptian art and architecture for millennia to come. Above all, he was a great physician, learned and kind, and the wider learning and practice of the humanities undoubtedly enhanced his qualities as a physician. When he died, Egypt wept; people lined the banks of the Nile in grief, as his body was taken down the river in a ceremonial barge. Egypt deified him as their God of medicine within a few generations of his demise.

Oh! What a difference between the age of Imhotep and the age of molecular biology, genetics and biotechnology. Yet, both are beautiful in their own way; both have their faults and blemishes—an age when science was non-existent, to an age where science dominates, to the extent that it demands evidence to shape the practice of clinical medicine. I refer to the oft-repeated mantra of evidence-based medicine. It is forgotten by physicians of today that some of the greatest benefits to mankind have been possible through simple observations, far removed from randomized, double-blind trials, and that much of medicine, whether we like it or not, is based on empiricism rather than on scientific proof.

Let me illustrate this fact by very briefly introducing some of our great predecessors in medicine.

We have Jenner who discovered the smallpox vaccination through a simple observation that those contacting cowpox were immune to smallpox. What greater benefit to humanity than the total eradication of smallpox—a disease that ravaged the world for centuries? Pasteur who enunciated the germ theory of medicine, stating that each disease is caused by a specific micro-organism and that a vaccine prepared from the specific organism could prevent the specific disease caused by the micro-organism; Semmelweiss who proved that doctors could by washing their hands sharply reduce the mortality of childbirth fever; Lister who discovered that dressing wounds with an antiseptic solution could prevent infection and who introduced the concept of asepsis in the practice of surgery; and Fleming who observed that a growth of staphylococci in a petri dish was decimated by the accidental growth of a fungus around the colonies of this bacterium. The active portion of the fungus responsible for this was identified as penicillin, the first antibiotic that could effect a cure in numerous hitherto fatal infections.

I need not go further in this list. Suffice it to say that you cannot understand the present nor anticipate the future if you are unaware of the past. T. S. Eliot grasps this instinctively when, in his poem 'The Four Quartets', he versifies—

Time present and time past
Are both perhaps present in time future
And time future contained in time past.

Why should an awareness and knowledge of history, not just medical history, but history viewed in a wider sense, be beneficial to a physician? Arnold Toynbee defines history as a study of civilizations. History to my mind is really a study of mankind and of all the existing factors that influence mankind over a period of time.

Now let us ask ourselves another question: what is medicine? Medicine is the study of man; man in the environment that surrounds him; man (so the ancients decreed) as a part of nature. We note the obvious overlap between the study of history and the study and practice of medicine. The poet Alexander Pope intuitively grasps this, when in his poem 'An Essay on Man', he versifies: 'The proper study of mankind is man'.

The concept that medicine is the study of man was initiated in the fifth century BCE by the Greek philosopher Pythagoras who founded the Italic School, off the southern coast of Italy. Pythagoras was the first to use the word 'philosophy'. According to the ancient Greeks, it was philosophy that determined the study of man in all his manifold aspects, with the express purpose of devising a healthy, satisfying, happy life. Medicine was for the first time being freed from its magico-religious beliefs and was invested with a rational basis.

Medicine, through the ages, has been influenced by philosophy, religion, economics, sociology, geography, art and culture; by conflicts, wars and natural disasters; and by the rise and fall of mighty empires. Above all, increasingly in the past hundred years, particularly in the past fifty years, it has been strongly, almost overpoweringly, influenced by the natural sciences. We cannot conceive of history to merely include governance, good or bad; to battles won and lost; or to the rise and fall of civilizations. It includes all the above and all that has influenced and continues to influence man and mankind. Amazingly, history has influenced both man and medicine, perhaps just as much as man and medicine have influenced history. The physician should not therefore view medicine with a narrow perspective. The historical evolution of medicine can only be understood against the tapestry of the civilization of man. A physician who is acquainted with the history of the world and who appreciates the various factors that have influenced man and medicine through the ages will understand his patient far better than one who is merely a master of the technicalities and science of medicine. He will have a more holistic view of his patient; he will have cultivated a better perception of health and disease and will not minister just to one or more dysfunctional organs, but to the patient as a whole. He will almost certainly be kinder, more compassionate, and will find it easier to strike an empathy with his patient, bonding the doctor–patient relationship that lies at the very heart of clinical medicine.

* * *

It was William Osler who said that the practising physician, and even the medical student, should have a bedside library. He included in his library Shakespeare, the Bible, Plutarch and Marcus Aurelius. I would further include the Bhagavad Gita, Rabindranath Tagore, Hemingway and Sir Arthur Conan Doyle. I am fascinated also with the Greek tragedies of Sophocles and Euripides. There is a bottomless treasure trove to choose from and place at one's bedside. Many schools in the West have established departments of medical humanities. These would result in shaping doctors with greater conscience, ethics, compassion and humility. I feel it unfortunate that admission to medical schools in our country is based on the knowledge of memorized imperfectly understood facts of science. It is time that our universities and colleges devise a curriculum or at least a course teaching medical humanities. A wider knowledge of humanities and of the universe we live in would perhaps be a far better background to help shape a good, discerning physician.

Let me elaborate a little on the value of the humanities to the practising physician by a few examples. The humanities include literature, poetry, ethics, religion, philosophy and social science. The humanities also include the arts—visual art, theatre, music and cinema. A study of the humanities develops in the physician an aesthetic sense, an inner refinement of spirit, a sensitivity and sensibility that shapes his conduct, and an acute awareness of the influence of the mind on human behaviour and of the mind on the mind–body complex. It helps the physician to improve his analytical and observational skills and inculcates a greater sense of ethical and moral values which will stand him in good stead in our fast changing world, where there seems to be a decline in values in almost all fields of human endeavour. Cultural and social beliefs govern an individual's experience of an illness, just as philosophy and religion condition his response and expectations. A physician who understands these issues is wiser by far.

The humanities also allow a deep insight into and an understanding of human nature and of the resilience and bravery often observed in the human spirit. They breed compassion and a sense of caring so that the physician regards his work as not just a profession but also a calling.

Literature, poetry, philosophy and religion give an in-depth insight into the meaning of suffering, both physical and mental. They teach the various ways in which human beings respond to suffering and how while pain and suffering often shatter the mind, body and spirit, they can yet be met with philosophical calm, and above all occasionally ignite the flame of creativity and genius in some talented individuals.

The world in the last instance is paradoxically rendered richer and more beautiful through suffering.

The relation between deep suffering and creativity is fascinating. I shall now lighten this discussion with a touch of poetry and philosophy. The poet Edna St Vincent Millay alternated between the intense mental suffering and darkness of depression and the overwhelming light and euphoria of mania. She described the feeling of depression and the lifting of darkness in beautiful verse in her poem 'Renascence', where at one point she says:

> How can I bear it; buried here,
> While overhead the sky grows clear

And then, later:

> And all at once the heavy night
> Fell from my eyes and I could see,—
> A drenched and dripping apple-tree

And then finally, we glimpse perhaps the euphoria of early mania, or is it just the expression of irrepressible relief?

> I raised my quivering arms on high;
> I laughed and laughed into the sky

Edna St Vincent committed suicide—note her premonition of the end when in her poem 'First Fig' she writes this—

> My candle burns at both ends;
> It will not last the night;
> But ah, my foes, and oh, my friends—
> It gives a lovely light!

Now listen to Emily Dickinson when threatened with blindness. She versified thus:

My loss, by sickness—was it Loss?
Or that Ethereal Gain
One earns by measuring the Grave—
Then—measuring the Sun—

The flowering of great inspiration and genius is best illustrated by Nietzsche who in the depths of despair and in deep physical and mental torment wrote one of his greatest works, *Thus Spake Zarathustra*, where he says:

Sing and bubble over, O Zarathustra, heal your soul with new songs, so that you may bear your great destiny. . . , *you are the teacher of the eternal recurrence*

He then goes on:

O man! Attend!
What does deep midnight's voice contend?
'I slept my sleep,
'And now awake at dreaming's end:
'The world is deep,
'And deeper than day can comprehend.
'Deep is its woe,
'Joy—deeper than its heart's agony:
'Woe says: Fade! Go!
'But all joy wants eternity,
'Wants deep, deep, deep eternity!'

Why have I dwelt at length on suffering? Because the physician meets suffering all the time. It wrenches his heart; he needs to relieve it. He needs to however know the inside of suffering, if he is to understand it well. He needs to know that suffering is conditioned by the patient's philosophy, religion, worldview and empathy with the physician. He also needs to know that though suffering and pain can shatter the human spirit, it can also occasionally light the flame of genius. What better teacher does a physician have to enable him to grasp suffering in its entirety than a study and love for the humanities?

A word about the understanding and appreciation of music: Music therapy to help healing has been in practice for several years. Music is the most evocative and, in my opinion, the most supreme, the greatest, of all art forms—it is indeed a blessing to man on earth. I have discussed this at length in my essay 'Music, the Mind and Medicine' later in this book.

I would like to summarize all that I have said earlier in a single sentence—*an awareness, knowledge and appreciation of history and the humanities, humanizes medicine.* The idea that history ought to serve medicine as a humanizing force has been a persistent refrain in discerning minds. Modern biomedicine for all its technical prowess is insufficient to produce good, caring physicians and caring healthcare systems. History and the humanities counterbalance the force of science. In his paper 'The Humanizing Power of Medical History', John Harley Warner says of history and the humanities—'They serve as a cohesive force binding medicine together in the face of the splintering tendencies of an increasingly specialized medical world'.

* * *

William Osler was the first to protest against the cultural impoverishment following the rise of science. The first chair of the Department of the History of Medicine was in fact established at Johns Hopkins Hospital in 1929. Later, Harvey Cushing, the neurosurgeon, took over this post. Let me quote Cushing in his speech at the inauguration of the American Osler Society in 1960:

In the modern development of the physician into a scientist have we not lost something precious that may without risk of pedantry be brought back to medicine? Not only has the art of healing—*die Heilkunst*—come more and more to be lost sight of as the doctor arrives at his diagnosis in the laboratory than at the bedside, but less and less does he care to be reminded that poetry, history, rhetoric, and the humanities had close kinship with natural philosophy when *Doctore Medicinae* took the lead among the *Artisti*.

The humanizing force exerted by the awareness of history and the humanities influences medicine by enhancing the art of medicine. It is the art of medicine that forms the final part of my essay.

Over a hundred years ago, William Osler said, 'Medicine is an art based on science. The practice of medicine is a science of uncertainty and an art of probability'. Since then there has been an explosion of knowledge, science and technology with reference to medicine. Even so, there remains a great degree of truth in his statement.

It is difficult to describe the art within medicine. For one, the art is intrinsically mixed with its science; for another, the art within medicine has no physical attributes but abstract qualities of the mind and heart, which blend to vibrate in empathy with an ill individual, contributing significantly to healing. Finally, it is an art that today has been pushed aside by the triumphs of modern science. It now lurks in the shadows, a forgotten art, perhaps in time to come, a lost art.

Let me quote Paracelsus, a great, renowned Renaissance physician: a physician must 'have the feel and touch which make it possible for him to be in sympathetic communication with the patient's spirit'. This last sentence epitomizes the intangible qualities that lie at the heart of medicine.

How does a doctor even begin to achieve this 'sympathetic communication' with a 'patient's spirit'? It is first and foremost by listening to the patient who seeks his or her help and taking a good history. Taking a patient's history is a forgotten art; yet a good history very often gives the diagnosis or offers a clue to the solution of a very difficult problem. The art of history-taking can never be perfectly mastered, even by the most accomplished physician. A disease often does not run true to type in that the same disease may manifest differently in different patients. Each patient is a unique individual; his response to disease may well be unique. This response depends not only on the disease process but also on the physiological alterations and the adaptations to physiological change; it is conditioned by the genetic make-up, the environment, constitution, physical endurance, emotional and mental state, and perhaps by several other unknown protean factors. Also, each patient interprets what happens to him or her in a unique way, and the expression in words to the doctor of what he or she feels can take different forms. For the doctor to be able to distinguish the relevant from the irrelevant, to separate the chaff from the grain, so as to touch the heart of the matter is indeed a challenging task.

What is the secret of a good history? First and foremost, it is listening to the patient, hearing him patiently and encouraging him to speak. Compare it to listening uninterruptedly to a raga or a piece of music. To listen effectively one must listen not just with the ears, but with one's whole self, with all of one's senses, for then only will a trained physician hear an unspoken problem. It is not enough to ferret the nature of a patient's disease; it is equally important while listening to assess the patient's emotional state, to get to know the province of his mind, which could either colour his disease or actually be responsible for his complaints.

After listening comes the art of questioning the patient. There are some patients who would agree with all a physician asks—they love to please the doctor. There are some who overplay one or more symptoms, only to deceive the doctor; there are others who are taciturn and who need to be coaxed gently, cleverly, to open up. They often underplay their symptoms and sometimes unwittingly hide the underlying seriousness of a life-threatening problem. And then there are some who mask their problems in a mass of irrelevant disconnected verbiage. A clue to their problems may lie buried within a plethora of words or in a sentence muttered as an aside.

The art of medicine is in assessing the patient as a whole—the mind and the body. Many patients come with complaints referred to an organ-system but whose true origin is due to a disturbance in the mind—the result of stress, worry, conflicts and frustrations that often plague modern existence. To fail to recognize this is to perpetuate the patient's problem, to order expensive tests that could be ruinous to the family, and to induce the patient to shop from doctor to doctor.

I need to express my thoughts on the importance of clinical judgement. A physician needs to be a judge. Judgement is indeed difficult, for medicine has been defined as the 'art of coming to a conclusion on insufficient evidence'. It is no surprise that errors in judgement frequently abound. Clinical judgement is a special quality, a faculty often inborn and occasionally cultivated. It cannot be equated to intellectual ability for it may be lacking in brilliant minds and be present to a marked degree in those who are far less clever or knowledgeable. It can only be cultivated or enhanced by a knowledge of history and the humanities, which gives an added dimension to medicine, enabling the physician to view medicine not through blinkers but to view it against the background of the tapestry of human civilization.

Clinical judgement requires more than factual knowledge, reason, logic, experience and skill. Clinical judgement is a rich blend of all of the above but involves a further intangible, indefinable quality—a quality that encompasses faith, charity, hope and compassion; a quality that has a deep understanding of human nature; a quality that can reach out to and sustain the shattered morale or the broken spirit of a seriously ill human being. It is also the quality that gives the doctor in a crisis the wisdom to know what to say and do and what not to say and do; when to wait and watch and when to treat vigorously without delay; when to fight death and when to give in to it; when to press for cure and when to console with words or to rest content with palliative relief. Good clinical judgement in a physician includes an extra-special perceptive ability to 'sense' a clue which his less fortunate colleagues will miss, the ability to process this clue and judge its correct diagnostic, therapeutic and prognostic implications.

A physician who combines the sharpness of his perceptive faculties with a wisdom born of experience and reading of history, literature, poetry, philosophy and religion—the humanities in brief—will be compassionate with a deep understanding of human suffering. He will also possess the faculty of good clinical judgement. Such a physician is truly blessed by the gods, for he has an attribute which no machine can duplicate and no science can invent. A physician with these attributes enjoys a ringside seat in the theatre of life. The world is a stage, and he has the most intimate insight into many who cross this stage and seek his help. He has the ability and the wisdom to alter for the better the drama of their lives.

* * *

Let me now attempt a definition of the art of medicine. The art of medicine lies in the artful application of its science to the overall holistic care of an individual patient. A physician steeped in the art knows the value of kindness, sympathy and caring in the healing of a patient. The art of medicine remains all-pervasive, even when its science fails or has reached its utmost limits. For when all the marvels of science are of no avail to unfortunately ward off the fatal end, then, as Dr Alfred Stille said, 'It is no small portion of [a physician's] art to rid his patient's path of thorns if he cannot make it bloom with roses'.

The art of medicine lies in hearing an unspoken, subtle nuance in a patient's history and in the ability to spot and appreciate the significance of one or more subtle physical signs that no gadget or machine could possibly recognize. It also lies in the ability of a physician to sift the evidence before him and give the right answer (of several possible answers) to the appropriate question. The art of medicine (even though the scientist might scoff) also lies in the intuitive feel for a solution either in diagnosis or management. Above all, it consists of looking at a sick patient holistically and in assessing not just the body but also the mind. The art of medicine is the art of healing, not just treating, not even just curing. Yet, it is only when art and science join hands that healing is best accomplished. It is only then that a physician can engage the unique individuality of a particular human being, thereby enabling him to assess not just the disease but the patient as a whole. A broader engagement between the doctor and the patient gives a holistic perspective, lends clarity to judgement and helps overcome the difficulties of decision-making. It bonds the doctor and the patient in a mutual trusting close-knit relationship that has stood the test of time.

Yes, it is an awareness of history and the humanities that ennobles the art, science and profession of medicine, just as it ennobles the profession of law, or for that matter, all other professions. The humanities (literature, poetry, music) cast their net figuratively speaking over humanity, as such promoting oneness among people and prompting, nay urging, the concern of one for the other. I am reminded of the famous lines of John Donne:

Each man's death diminishes me,
For I am involved in mankind.
Therefore, send not to know
For whom the bell tolls,
It tolls for thee.

History enriches not just medicine but the world. As Winston Churchill said: 'History with its flickering lamp stumbles along the trail of the past, trying to reconstruct its scenes, to revive its echoes, and kindle with pale gleams the passion of former days.' In Greek mythology, the guardian of Time was a two-headed god called Janus. With one head he looked at the past and gave the wisdom of his hindsight to man, with the other head he looked into the future and if there was a man brave enough to step forward into the unknown, he gave him the benefit of his foresight. Yes, ladies and gentlemen, to put it in Churchill's words, 'The further backward you can look, the further forward you can see'.

2

The Fight against Infection

The Microbe Hunters

In the nineteenth century, men lost their fear of God and acquired a fear of microbes.

—ANONYMOUS

The middle of the nineteenth century witnessed a great landmark in the history of man and medicine—the coming of age of the science of bacteriology and microbiology. This science and those who pioneered it brought about a true revolution in medicine. It was a revolution that finally resolved age-old controversies on the cause of infections and infectious diseases, and it came about when, after 1860, medical researchers began to prove that infections were caused by micro-organisms—living organisms that invaded the body with devastating results. It is tempting to compare the far-reaching effects of this nineteenth-century revolution in medicine with the French Revolution of 1789. The first drastically altered the face of medicine; the second shattered the sociopolitical framework of France and was a prelude to similar changes in other countries of the West.

Until the middle of the nineteenth century, infected wounds and other infections were responsible for great morbidity and a forbiddingly high mortality. In fact, the chief cause of morbidity and mortality after surgery was infection. Surgical wards were like charnel houses. Gangrene often complicated injuries and wounds; it also was a dreadful complication following amputation and other surgical procedures. It often raged like an epidemic in surgical wards, whose air was foul and foetid with the stink of festering wounds and rotting flesh. Secondary haemorrhage subsequent to infected wounds, post-operative tetanus and septicaemia contributed further to mortality. The soldier in the battlefield almost certainly had a better chance to survive in battle than a patient in his ordeal consequent to surgery.

Infectious diseases were also rampant, often in epidemic form. These included smallpox, plague, cholera, typhoid, typhus, tetanus, malaria and several other diseases. These diseases—in particular smallpox, cholera and plague—struck at frequent intervals, decimating mankind all over the world, almost since the beginning of the history of man. The cause of infections till this period of man's history was a hotbed of controversy and dispute. The generally accepted view was that disease (and this included infections as the major cause of disease) was due to 'miasmas', 'humours', or 'vapours' or even the presence of oxygen in the air.

A few visionaries challenged the miasmic theory of the cause of disease as early as the Renaissance. The contagiousness of infectious diseases such as plague, smallpox, diphtheria, cholera, typhoid and syphilis, which could spread like wildfire through countries, was long felt to be due to the passing of infection from infected individuals to others. As early as 1546, Girolamo Fracastoro had postulated that *seminaria contagiosa* ('seeds of disease') from infected patients could produce disease in uninfected individuals through direct contact. In the early nineteenth century, Agostino Bassi of Lodi was among the first to suggest the relation between micro-organisms and disease. He studied *mal del segno*, a silkworm disease, and observed that it was caused by a living organism, *Botrytis paradoxa*. He observed white marks on the bodies of the affected worms and concluded that silkworm disease was caused by a living vegetable parasite. On the basis of many other experiments, Bassi asserted in 1846 that disease was not caused by humours but by a living organism—an animal or vegetable parasite. He thus anticipated the cause of infectious disease so ably discovered and enunciated by Louis Pasteur ten years later.

The controversies on the theories of infection also involved theories of putrefaction and decomposition of organic matter, such as food, vegetable matter and meat. The presence of insects, mites and other organisms in decaying matter was a recognized feature of putrefaction. The origin of these living organisms was however in dispute. There were some who believed in the theory that the putrefaction of matter produced these organisms by 'spontaneous generation'; there were others who maintained that it was pre-existing living organisms that were responsible for decay and putrescence. Lazzaro Spallanzani of Italy, for example, disbelieved the theory of spontaneous generation. He maintained that broth, if boiled and then hermetically sealed, would keep indefinitely without generating any living organisms. There were metaphysical and philosophical overtones to the arguments for and against the theory of spontaneous generations.

Friedrich Gustav Jacob Henle of Germany was among the first to declare that infectious diseases were not caused by humours or miasmas but by living micro-organisms, which acted as parasites on entering the body. He debunked the theory of miasmas in infections and of spontaneous generation in putrefaction. He also postulated that once the causative organisms of disease were discovered, cure should follow. Henle's views were speculative, and the debate in relation to the causes and mechanisms of infection continued unabated. Like Fracastoro, Henle too believed in seeds of disease and postulated that these could be carried by the wind and infect even individuals who were not in direct contact with infected patients. But then, what were these 'seeds of disease'? What was their form and structure, where did they originate, and how did they cause disease in mankind? Fracastoro indeed had a great prophetic vision but a vision that remained veiled and shrouded in mystery for three hundred years.

The man who first disproved the theory of poisonous vapours in relation to infections by careful prolonged observation and study was the Hungarian obstetrician Ignaz Philipp Semmelweis (1818–65). It was however Louis Pasteur, perhaps the greatest research scientist France has ever produced, and Robert Koch, an equally great research scientist in Germany, who in the middle and latter half of the nineteenth century scientifically proved that the seeds of disease postulated by Fracastoro in the Renaissance period were living micro-organisms. Their work rang the death-knell to the miasmatic theory of disease.

While this background is important for context, this essay is mainly concerned with the seminal observations on childbirth fever by Semmelweis, the great scientific discoveries of Pasteur and Koch, and the introduction of antisepsis and asepsis in surgery by Joseph Lister. Pasteur and Koch opened the door to a host of other scientists and researchers, introducing medicine to the world of micro-organisms—a world within a world, a hitherto unknown, invisible world that co-exists on this planet with man.

* * *

Ignaz Philipp Semmelweis demolished the theory of poisonous vapours without being aware as to what caused infections. This was indeed a remarkable scientific achievement. He qualified from the University of Vienna in 1844. Two years later, he joined the first maternity ward of the Vienna Krankenhaus as assistant to Professor Johann Klein, a famous obstetrician. In that era, infections and severe sepsis were equally frequent in mothers after childbirth. This infection called childbirth fever (now termed puerperal sepsis) also carried a tragic mortality. In 1840, the mortality of childbirth in this famous maternity clinic was forbiddingly high. Semmelweis was increasingly distressed at the many deaths among the mothers in his maternity ward, which in the first year was close to 40 per cent. He searched for clues for this high mortality and discovered that the mortality rate in the second maternity ward was four to five times less. It was highly improbable that poisonous vapours could selectively kill mothers in the first maternity ward. He had also noted that in the first maternity ward where the mortality was high, doctors attended to the mothers after delivery, whereas in the second maternity ward with a low mortality rate, midwives were in charge. He then made a shrewd observation that connected the autopsy room to the high maternal mortality in his ward. It was customary for obstetricians to start the day by first carrying out autopsies on the mothers under their care who had died after childbirth and then proceed with their ward work. The midwives looking after the second maternity ward never attended autopsies. Semmelweis was convinced that early morning visits to the autopsy room by the doctors of his ward were responsible for the high maternal mortality. He felt that the low mortality in the ward managed by the midwives was because the midwives never entered the autopsy room.

This conviction was born in 1847, when Semmelweis went for a short holiday to Venice. On his return, he was saddened to learn of the death of his colleague Jakob Kolletschka, who was assistant to the great pathologist Karl Rokitansky. Kolletschka had died after a scalpel wound sustained while performing an autopsy on a mother who had died of childbirth fever. Semmelweis attended the autopsy of his friend and was shocked to observe that the lesions in various organ systems were very similar to those observed in mothers dying of childbirth fever. The scalpel had unquestionably transferred infection from the corpse to his poor friend. Semmelweis was convinced that infections in the maternity ward were conveyed to mothers by doctors who performed autopsies and then immediately visited the maternity ward to examine mothers and help in childbirth. Semmelweis now gave strict instructions that the wards were to be cleaned with calcium chloride and that before touching a patient, everyone was to wash their hands thoroughly and then dip them in an antiseptic solution of calcium chloride. This elementary precaution resulted in a sharp decline in the mortality rate of mothers, which went down to nearly zero within two years. Semmelweis communicated these findings to the medical society in Vienna, claiming that puerperal sepsis or childbirth fever was a form of blood poisoning or septicaemia that was transmitted to mothers by unwashed contaminated hands, and that the simple precaution of washing hands and dipping them in a reliable antiseptic sharply reduced the incidence of this dreadful infection. His observations and his views were sharply attacked by all obstetricians and also by almost the whole medical faculty. There were, however, three great professors who agreed with him and staunchly supported him. They were the great pathologist Karl Rokitansky; the great physician Josef Skoda, famed for his diagnostic ability and for pioneering the use of percussion and auscultation in Austria; and the dermatologist Ferdinand Ritter von Hebra.

The obstetricians of the Vienna Krankenhaus, however, ganged up against Semmelweis, and he was forced to resign.

A saddened, frustrated Semmelweis returned to his native Budapest. Doctors and students at the Vienna Krankenhaus stopped washing and disinfecting their hands, and the mortality rate in delivered mothers soared to its original high level. In Budapest, Semmelweis became head of obstetrics at St Rochus Hospital and continued to practise antisepsis in his maternity wards. Not only did he insist on handwashing but also insisted that all instruments and dressings be disinfected, that fresh linen be provided for each patient, and that the wards be periodically disinfected. Maternal mortality dipped sharply and puerperal sepsis seemed a nightmare of the past.

The rest of this great man's tragic life was spent in his trying to convince the world that the simple act of handwashing could save thousands of lives. He published his beliefs and his work in *Die Ätiologie, der Begriff und die Prophylaxe des Kindbettfiebers* (The Cause, Concept and Prophylaxis of Childbirth Fever) in 1881. It was an epoch-making landmark in the history of medicine. Its message was direct, simple, and had far-reaching consequences. Yet, the reaction to the book was extremely hostile. Europe rejected Semmelweis' views; the medical profession scorned his work. Rudolf Virchow, the greatest name in pathology in the mid-nineteenth century, refuted Semmelweis' observations and conclusions. Semmelweis was further embittered, and when he visited one of his few friends Ferdinand Ritter von Hebra in Vienna in 1864, he showed signs of mental instability. He was finally kept in a mental asylum, where he died within a few weeks.

There are many today who consider Ignaz Philipp Semmelweis as one of the greatest medical benefactors of humanity. His life was a dark, tragic struggle, during which he made a great contribution to medicine. His views, today, have assumed even greater relevance. Handwashing is considered to be the single most important feature in the prevention of nosocomial infections in hospitals, particularly in critical care units. There now stands a monument in Budapest to mark the memory of this great man. It was constructed twenty-nine years after his death in 1894, perhaps to atone for the way the world treated him when he was alive. His everlasting tribute, posthumous though this may be, stems from the benefits he conferred on humanity. What greater tribute could a man of medicine ever wish for?

* * *

Around the middle of the nineteenth century, there strode on the stage of history a great man—Louis Pasteur. He was a chemist, not a doctor, yet he unravelled the mystery of infection with a surety that stopped all debate and opened up a glorious vista for science, medicine, and for the benefit of man. If one were to list the ten great scientists and researchers in medicine, Pasteur would surely be among the list.

Before discussing Pasteur, his discoveries, and the discoveries of those who followed him, it is relevant to briefly touch upon the instrument that made their work possible. This instrument was the microscope, which enabled the scientist to magnify very small objects invisible to the naked eye. The advent of the microscope was an important milestone; it ushered a new era both in the natural sciences and medicine. In all probability, Johannes and Zacharias Jansen of Middleburg in Holland invented the microscope in 1590. However, Anton van Leeuwenhoek (1632–1723), who has erroneously been described as the microscope's inventor, significantly modified the instrument for the better.

Leeuwenhoek was an amateur who had no formal education but was brilliant in innovations and inventions and was seized by an unquestionable curiosity to search for the truth. He was a draper born in Delft, Holland. He had never left his native city, never visited a university and knew no language other than Dutch. He first used the lens in his business to count the threads of fabric. He personally made over four hundred microscopes, improving the instrument so that he ultimately achieved a magnification up to 200 times. He spent hours at the microscope looking upon animate and inanimate objects. He wrote amusingly that he saw under his microscope graceful little animals more numerous than all the inhabitants of the Low Countries when he examined a piece of food found between his teeth. Thus, a humble uneducated draper showed for the first time that the ecological environment of man also included extremely minute organisms invisible to the naked eye. Even though Leeuwenhoek proved that micro-organisms (organisms invisible to the naked eye) existed, the relation between humans, their ecology, and infection remained unsolved. The microscope underwent further improvement and was aptly refined, contributing a great deal to the advances in microbiology. It was the sword used by Pasteur and many who followed him in the fight against infection.

* * *

Louis Pasteur was born in Dole in the French district of Jura on 27 December 1822. He was the son of a tanner who had served as a sergeant in Napoleon's Grande Armée. Pasteur first went to college at Besançon and then went on to Paris at the École normale supérieure, where he graduated in chemistry. His first love was chemistry. He exhibited from the start a clarity and brilliance of thought and ideas, a flair for laboratory work, a meticulousness in experimentation and observation, and a refined logic to his many discoveries that would rank him as the greatest man of the nineteenth century.

Pasteur's early work was in chemistry—the study of polarization of light by tartaric acid crystals. He demonstrated that molecular asymmetry in the tartaric acid crystals governed the behaviour of light and concluded that this molecular asymmetry distinguished inanimate forms from animate or living beings. This work led to the development of stereochemistry. In 1852, Pasteur became a professor of chemistry at the University of Strasbourg, and two years later, he moved on to the University of Lille. His interest now moved from chemistry to biology, from the study of crystals to the unravelling of the mystery of living micro-organisms and their relation to mankind and disease. In his inaugural lecture at the University of Lille, he made a profound statement that was indeed very apt in relation to his many discoveries: 'In the field of observation, chance favours only the prepared mind'. His time had come; he was by now prepared to embark on his voyage of discovery. In 1857, he was appointed Director of Scientific Studies at the École normale supérieure, and from that point in time, his destiny was to be fulfilled.

Let me first briefly encompass Pasteur's study on micro-organisms unrelated to infections in humans. Indeed, there was an extremely vital prelude to his subsequent work on the relation between the role of micro-organisms in the causation of infectious diseases. He postulated and solved the following contentious issues that prevailed at this time. I shall not go into details of the work, but rest content by summarizing this work for the reader.

Pasteur proved that fermentation was a biological process caused by specific living micro-organisms. He convincingly demolished the widely held belief that fermentation was caused by the chemical breakdown of dead yeast. He showed that living organisms brought about the decomposition of wine with the production of vinegar, and that milk would decompose into lactic acid under the influence of lactic acid bacilli. He called this process 'fermentation' when the end product was useful and 'putrefaction' when it was harmful.

He then went on to discover bacilli responsible for butyric acid fermentation. He noted that these bacilli could live without oxygen and flourished in an atmosphere of carbon dioxide. He named these 'anaerobic organisms'—in contrast to 'aerobic organisms', which required oxygen to live and multiply.

He finally demonstrated through an elegant system of experiments that the theory of spontaneous generation of organisms as the cause of putrefaction was untenable. An ardent supporter of spontaneous generation in France was Félix Pouchet, who based his theory on his own experiments. Pasteur contended that Pouchet's experiments suffered from faulty technique and thus led to incorrect conclusions. His counter-experiments proved the immediate and essential role of micro-organisms in putrefaction. France followed the usual custom of setting up a court of inquiry into debatable scientific issues. The French Académie des Sciences decided to adjudicate between Pasteur and Pouchet in the theory of putrefaction. After listening to arguments on both sides they pronounced the verdict in Pasteur's favour. The theory of spontaneous generation was thus buried for eternity by Louis Pasteur.

In 1864, France suffered an economic industrial disaster. Wine production from grapes was one of the chief industries of France, but wine producers were disturbed by the frequent souring of wine, which led to a great loss of revenue. They approached Pasteur for help and requested him to suggest a remedy. Pasteur researched on this subject and found that the organism *Mycetum aceti* was responsible for the fermentation of wine into sour vinegar. He discovered that bacteria-free fluids would remain sterile and free of organisms if properly protected. One way of protection was heat. He showed that heating wine for a short while to 60°C (140°F) killed the *Mycetum aceti* responsible for the fermentation to vinegar without spoiling the quality of wine. Protection of sterility through heat was applied to other liquids, e.g., milk, and came to be known as 'pasteurization', in honour of the man who first discovered this practice.

In 1865, the silk industry, another important industry in France, was nearly crippled and ruined by a disease called pébrine, which was destroying silkworms. Pasteur determined that the cause of silkworm disease was a living protozoan present in moths, their ova and the worms. He worked out the life cycle of this protozoan and showed that removing the infected ova prevented the spread of disease.

* * *

As mentioned earlier, these achievements were preludes to Pasteur's annunciation of his germ theory in 1868 to the French Academy of Medicine. In a joint paper with Jules Joubert (1824–1907) and Charles Chamberland (1851–1908), Pasteur contended that micro-organisms were responsible for infectious diseases, putrefaction and fermentation; that specific micro-organisms produced specific diseases. He concluded that if these micro-organisms could be identified then specific vaccines could be prepared and could well prevent specific diseases.

This was a brilliant hypothesis, largely intuitive, though at least in part, based on Pasteur's earlier work on micro-organisms. It revolutionized medicine in that era. He now needed to prove this hypothesis, and he did so in a brilliant fashion. In 1879, he had the chance to put his ideas to a practical test. Chicken cholera was raging in several areas of France. He identified the organisms and isolated them in pure culture. He then noted that old cultures lost their virulence, and poultry infected with these old cultures were protected when subsequently live virulent cultures were injected into them. He thus showed that poultry infected by old avirulent cultures were immunized and remained protected from contacting chicken cholera. His idea of protection from disease through vaccination was a brilliant thought, and he was proved right.

Next, Pasteur turned his attention to anthrax, a highly contagious disease affecting horses, cattle, and other ruminants and spreading to humans through contact with infected hides or meat. The death of livestock from anthrax was great, and the disease was particularly ruinous to this industry because it persisted and recurred in fields from which infected animals had been removed. In man, the disease produced necrotizing skin lesions or a fulminant fatal pneumonia. Franz Anton Aloys Pollender (1799–1879) and Casimir Joseph Davaine (1812–82) had found the anthrax bacillus in the blood of cattle dying of anthrax. Robert Koch, a great bacteriologist, was also studying anthrax around this time and had noted that under certain conditions the bacillus assumed the form of heat-resistant spores. These heat-resistant spores could contaminate the soil of fields and when they reverted to the bacillary form could produce disease. The persistence of anthrax in previously infected fields was thus proven by Koch to be related to the persistent presence of these spores.

Pasteur experimented with ways and means of reducing the virulence of the anthrax bacillus. He finally observed that the virulence was markedly decreased by heating the bacillus to 42°C (107°F). When these bacilli with attenuated virulence were now injected into normal sheep, the vaccinated sheep did not develop the disease when subsequently virulent bacilli were injected into them. Pasteur must have been a remarkable showman, indeed a rare trait for a scientist of such great genius. He resolved to give a public demonstration of the efficacy of the anthrax vaccine on 5 May 1881 at Pouilly-le-Fort near Melun. He took forty-eight sheep as the subjects of his study. Before a large crowd of farmers, journalists, veterinary surgeons and onlookers, he injected virulent anthrax bacilli into twenty-four sheep previously immunized by his anthrax vaccine and into twenty-four healthy sheep not immunized by his vaccine. After forty-eight hours, all the vaccinated sheep remained unaffected and well; twenty-two of the twenty-four unvaccinated sheep had died of anthrax.

* * *

Although crippled by a stroke that paralysed his right side, Pasteur now moved into his last great field of research—the prevention of rabies. This was and remains a dreadful disease characterized by hydrophobia, severe agitation and paralysis followed by certain death in a few days. It remains as fatal today as it was in antiquity. Pasteur first attempted to identify the organism causing rabies; he failed, not surprisingly, since the disease is caused by a virus only visible through an electron microscope. He noted, however, that in dogs with rabies, the infecting organism was present not only in saliva but also in the spinal cord. He began injecting spinal cord tissue containing the infective organism into rabbit brains. When one rabbit after another had been injected with this virus, a fixed incubation period of six days was observed. He called the virus acting in this manner a *virus fixe*. He injected this virus into the spinal cord of rabbits and after their death, dried the spinal cord. On drying the cord for two weeks, he observed that the virus was well-nigh non-virulent. In 1884, Pasteur made fourteen graduated vaccines of increasing potency. He injected the vaccine daily for fourteen days into normal healthy dogs, starting with the weakest and graduating to the strongest, thereby conferring immunity to rabies on these dogs. When these immunized dogs were challenged with the rabies virus after fourteen days they remained healthy. When the same virus was injected into healthy non-immunized dogs, they all succumbed. This in itself was an immense achievement. What prompted him to experiment in the manner described above can never be explained. It points to his ingenuity and intuitive grasp of not just the problem but also its solution, as also of his brilliance in experimental medicine. To succeed in making a vaccine protecting dogs from rabies even when the cause or the micro-organism causing the disease was in that day and age not identified seems a stupendous feat. Pasteur demonstrated to a government commission the efficacy of this anti-rabies vaccine in protecting dogs from rabies. The question was, could the anti-rabies vaccine prevent rabies in humans bitten by rabid animals? Pasteur felt that it could, and he waited eagerly for an opportunity to try the vaccine on humans.

The day of judgement was soon to come. In the summer of 1885, Joseph Meister, a nine-year-old boy from Alsace, was bitten several times by a rabid dog. His doctor advised the boy's mother to take him to Pasteur. Ten days after coming to him and twelve days after the rabid dog's bites, Pasteur took the risk of vaccinating the young boy with his anti-rabies vaccine. The vaccine was given intramuscularly every day for fourteen days, starting with the weakest dose on the first day and slowly graduating to the strongest dose on the fourteenth day. Pasteur must have waited with bated breath. The risk was immense; the suspense, almost unbearable. Taking a risk of such magnitude could have only stemmed from an invincible courage based on strong conviction. Yet, imagine the opprobrium, the tragedy, the inglorious end to a brilliant scientific career, if Joseph Meister had died of rabies following Pasteur's experiment. But Pasteur was a man born to a great destiny. Joseph Meister—to what must have been Pasteur's intense joy and relief—mercifully lived, and stayed healthy. What is more, three months after Joseph Meister sought his help, another victim came to Pasteur's door. He was a fourteen-year-old shepherd from Pasteur's home district of Jura. He had been badly bitten while trying to save others from the attack of a rabid dog. Pasteur vaccinated him in the same manner, and this boy also survived. On 26 October 1885, Pasteur wrote to the French Académie des Sciences that Joseph Meister was safe and well.

The story of this human drama between Pasteur, Joseph Meister and the prevention of rabies took the world by storm. Anti-rabies vaccination, as discovered by Pasteur, became the standard procedure all over the world in the prevention of rabies. This indeed was a magnificent finale, the crowning glory of an incredibly great career. Pasteur symbolized the quintessential spirit of science and scientific inquiry. To the world, he was a great hero; every discovery he made had led to the benefit of mankind. Perhaps no man of science has been so greatly and so universally honoured as Louis Pasteur. The Institut Pasteur was set up in 1888 to enable him to continue his research on micro-organisms and on the development of specific vaccines against diseases. There, he gathered around him some of the most famous names in science who worked with him and who shared his travails and joys. Yet, we must remember that it was not a man who studied and trained in medicine, but a chemist who ranks as one of the greatest benefactors of mankind. It is said that a French newspaper put out a questionnaire to its readers as to who they considered the greatest Frenchman of all time. Pasteur, not surprisingly, received even more votes than Napoleon and Charlemagne. Pasteur died at the age of seventy-two in 1895. The Institut Pasteur remains to this day a living monument to his name and fame; many renowned scientists have followed his footsteps in the sands of time.

* * *

While Semmelweis was working in Vienna devising methods to reduce the horrendous mortality in childbirth fever, and Pasteur in Paris was researching micro-organisms and their relation to diseases, Joseph Lister was working in Scotland and breaking new ground in the field of surgery. Lister was an excellent surgeon, a surgeon who did not equate the art and science of surgery merely with dexterity and speed. He was a thinking surgeon, deeply concerned all through his life with unsolved surgical problems confronting him. Two great landmarks in surgery stand to his name. He showed how to prevent infection in wounds, and more importantly, he introduced the concept of asepsis in surgery—a concept that was non-existent before his time, but because of him, is today the very bedrock of surgical practice.

The child is the father of man, and Lister's early background may well have shaped and tempered his scientific career.

His father, Joseph Jackson Lister, was a scientist who had made significant contributions to the improvement of the microscope. Young Lister was thus in close contact from his early days with the spirit of scientific enquiry. His parents, who imparted the principles of plain living and high thinking, were from a Quaker background. As a young boy, Lister was hardworking but had to be taken away from school for a short time for what was probably a nervous breakdown. This boyhood crisis may well harbour some of the secrets of the personality traits of this great man. Lister was often painfully shy, afflicted by a stammer, could never lecture without notes, and even after days of preparation would continue to work on these notes even as his carriage drove him to the lecture hall. He found it difficult to face an audience and, surprisingly for an Englishman, often kept his audience waiting by not arriving at the appointed time.

Lister graduated from University College, London, and continued his postgraduate studies at the same college. He was made a Fellow of the Royal College of Surgeons in 1852 and then went to study under the famous surgeon James Syme in Edinburgh, who was one of the best surgeons of his time. He soon became assistant surgeon to Syme at the Royal Infirmary. After six years of work in Edinburgh, Lister was appointed to the Regius Chair of Surgery in Glasgow. From the very start of his medical career, Lister grappled with the problem of infection of surgical wounds. Surgical wards in that era were filled with patients suffering from infected wounds, which suppurated, turned gangrenous and caused certain death. All through his work in London and Edinburgh, Lister attempted to determine the nature of inflammation, its cause, and measures to prevent inflammation graduating to suppuration and gangrene. He looked at some of the grey gangrenous matter under a microscope and made sketches of what he saw; he understood the pathology of inflammation, but there was no method to counter the progress of infection.

Then came the breakthrough. Very soon after he became the Professor of Surgery at Glasgow, darkness was dispelled by light. One day in 1865, when Lister was walking towards the surgical wards, his colleague Thomas Anderson, a professor of chemistry at the University of Glasgow, thrust a paper written by Louis Pasteur in Lister's hands. It was titled 'Recherches sur la putréfaction' (Research on Putrefaction). Pasteur wrote in his paper that putrefaction resulted from invisible micro-organisms suspended in the air. This revelation triggered the genius in Lister, enabling him to make a profound discovery. He argued that it must be these very organisms present in abundance in the air of the operating rooms and in surgical wards that caused infection, inflammation, suppuration, putrefaction and gangrene. He realized that microbes could be carried on surgical instruments, sponges, in clean wounds, and on surgeons' hands. The secret of success was to get rid of these micro-organisms by a suitable chemical antiseptic dressing until such time as the edges of the wound healed. Experience taught him that the smallest wound was vulnerable until it had completely healed.

Lister now introduced meticulous cleanliness in his ward and tried out numerous antiseptic solutions. Once again a fortuitous incident shaped his work. The town of Carlisle around this time had faced a disaster due to the seepage of sewage into adjacent pastures; this had resulted in the poisoning and death of many cattle grazing on these pastures. The problem had been rectified by the treatment of sewage with German creosote, which was an impure form of carbolic acid. Lister concluded that carbolic acid could kill bacteria and was eager to try its effect on preventing infection in wounds.

It was a common observation in surgery that a simple fracture of a long bone healed well without complicating infection. Yet a compound fracture, which is characterized by a clear break in the continuity of skin, always resulted in infection, suppuration and, very frequently, gangrene. In fact, the treatment of compound fractures in that age was amputation, for fear of gangrene setting in. Lister resolved to try the effect of carbolic acid on compound fractures. In March 1865, a factory worker had a severe compound fracture of the leg. Lister smeared carbolic acid over the lacerated wound; the patient died of shock from the injury before the carbolic acid treatment could show a conclusive result. Then at last, after years of infructuous struggle came the success story.

On 12 August 1865, an eleven-year-old boy was run over by an empty cart and suffered a compound fracture of both bones of the leg. There was a small open wound, which Lister dressed with a piece of lint soaked in carbolic acid. The bones were then set. This dressing was kept in place for four days; the wound remained free of infection. The boy made a good recovery. Lister now developed a specific method for the treatment of wounds. He used forceps to introduce a piece of lint soaked in carbolic acid into the wound, then covered the wound with a second piece of lint soaked in carbolic acid. He placed tinfoil on top to prevent evaporation of the antiseptic, and packed absorbent wool around the wound.

Before an operation, Lister sprayed the operation theatre with carbolic acid, spraying the instruments and also the patient's skin. During the operation, the air continued to be sprayed with carbolic acid, soaking all those present. The technique involved antisepsis, i.e., killing all micro-organisms in the wound, and asepsis, i.e., preventing bacteria from entering the wound. He published his successful results of compound fractures in the *Lancet* in 1867. None of his eleven compound fracture patients had died. He concluded in this paper that 'the element of incurability has been eliminated', a modest statement, its correct interpretation being that his discoveries had saved many lives.

Lister's theory of antisepsis and asepsis was ultimately widely accepted all over Europe and America. He achieved an iconic stature—surgeons from all over the world learnt from him and paid him homage. He rose to be the Chief of Surgery in Edinburgh and, in 1877, was appointed professor of surgery at King's College, London. Numerous honours were conferred on him by his own country and by countries all over the world. Yet, what greater honour can one ever hope for other than the gratitude of the very many whose lives one has helped to save? His eightieth birthday was celebrated all over the Western world; he remained at home listening to the stream of people who paid him their respects.

Lister died on 10 February 1912. London witnessed a great funeral at Westminster Abbey, but he was buried according to his wish at West Hampstead beside his wife Agnes. Agnes was the daughter of Professor Syme of Edinburgh, Lister's mentor. Lister had married her when he worked as assistant to Professor Syme. They were an extremely devoted couple, and Lister was emotionally shattered after her unfortunate death.

In his poem 'The Chief', the poet William Earnest Henley, who had been Lister's patient, wrote of him:

We hold him for another Herakles,
Battling with custom, prejudice, disease,
As once the son of Zeus with Death and Hell.

There are some important observations one can make with regard to these three greats in medicine—Semmelweis, Pasteur and Lister. Amazingly, none of them ever met. Perhaps they were not aware of each other's existence; they were certainly unaware of each other's work. When Lister married Professor Syme's daughter Agnes, he went on his honeymoon to various medical centres. These included Vienna, but he remained unaware of Semmelweis's work on childbirth fever. Had he met Semmelweis, his work on antisepsis and asepsis might have culminated earlier than it did. Finally, would Lister have stumbled upon the theory of antisepsis and asepsis in surgery if Thomas Anderson, the chemistry professor in Glasgow, had failed to give him Pasteur's work on putrefaction? Perhaps yes, but it would have taken much longer.

* * *

We must now consider the contribution of the great German scientist Robert Koch who indeed was a renowned microbe hunter. What Pasteur was to France, Koch was to Germany. Germany was immensely proud of his prowess as a scientist, and rightly so. Koch qualified in medicine in 1866 at the University of Gottingen. Remarkably enough, his initiation into medicine was as a surgeon in the Franco-Prussian war in which France suffered a crushing defeat. He then became a district officer in Wollstein, a small town in Prussia. Anthrax was prevalent in this area, and Koch in a makeshift laboratory succeeded in unravelling the bacteriology of this disease. He isolated the anthrax bacillus from the spleen of a dead animal, grew it on culture and worked out its full life history.

Koch developed great technical expertise and dexterity in laboratory work, contributing a great deal to the technical advances in the laboratory studies of bacteriology. These technical advances have stood the test of time and are of use even today. They include special staining and microscopic studies for the identification and study of bacteria, making use of the oil immersion lens. Koch also devised various media for the culture of specific organisms.

Unquestionably, Koch's greatest work and triumph was the discovery that tuberculosis was caused by a specific organism, *Mycobacterium tuberculosis*. This indeed was a unique achievement. René Laennec had described the clinical features of tuberculosis, which could not only involve the lungs but also many other organs. He had identified the 'tubercle', a macroscopic hallmark of tuberculosis involving various organs. Jean Antoine Villemin had described the pathology of tuberculous lesions and had demonstrated that the disease could be transmitted to animals by the injection of tuberculous material. Yet, the cause of tuberculosis, which had a high incidence and mortality in the Western world in the nineteenth century had not been discovered. Koch not only identified the organism causing tuberculosis but also succeeded in culturing it.

He presented his results in 1884 to the Berlin Physiological Society. He also presented in this paper his famous Koch's postulates, announcing a scientific discipline that needs to be fulfilled if a specific organism is to be responsible for a specific disease. His postulates were: (i) that the organism had to be always found in a given disease; (ii) that it was to be never found in other diseases or in health; (iii) that the organism must be grown on culture and that an injection of a pure culture in a susceptible animal must reproduce the disease; and (iv) that the organism must be present in the animal so innoculated.

One more important discovery of Koch is the discovery of the *Vibrio cholerae* that caused the epidemic disease cholera. The discovery of cholera is interesting. A cholera epidemic broke out in Egypt, and Koch was sent to investigate the disease. Also investigating the same problem was a French team headed by Pasteur's colleague, Pierre Paul Émile Roux. Roux followed Pasteur's method, which was to reproduce the disease in an animal and then identify the organism. Roux did not realize that cholera only occurred in humans and not in animals. He therefore failed. Koch looked out for the organism in infected stools and discovered *Vibrio cholerae* as the cause of the disease. Koch then went on to Calcutta (now Kolkata) where the disease was rife and showed that the organism lived in the intestine and that the disease spread through the contamination of water. There was indeed jubilation in Germany; the Germans felt that they had the equal of Louis Pasteur.

There is an amusing aside to this story. Though the miasmatic theory of disease was by now buried forever, there were some diehards who refused to believe that *Vibrio cholerae* caused cholera. Herr Doctor Pettenkofer of Munich was one such diehard. He requested Herr Doctor Professor Koch to send him a flask containing a pure culture of *Vibrio cholerae*. Koch obliged, whereupon Herr Doctor Pettenkofer swallowed (with relish) the contents of the flask. He wrote to Koch that he was in perfect health—where was the cholera? Perhaps Herr Doctor Pettenkofer's stomach had an unusually high acid content that destroyed the organisms, or perhaps the pure culture he swallowed had lost its virulence!

The economic and political rivalry between France and Germany in the last trimester of the nineteenth century was intense. Unfortunately, this crept surreptitiously into science—particularly the science of bacteriology. Koch probably felt the need to make one more great discovery that would eclipse Pasteur. He felt that this discovery had to be in relation to tuberculosis, which in that era was the scourge of the world. Could he not research and find the cure for this disease? He would then be immortalized for eternity.

Koch set to work in his laboratory and in August 1890, at the International Congress in Berlin, announced that he had discovered a substance that arrested the growth of the tubercle bacillus both in animals and humans. He called his substance 'tuberculin'. There was instant euphoria in the world. The world smiled; it had to be true! How could the great Robert Koch be wrong? Germany was seized with joyous frenzy. Koch was the hero of Germany. Germany heaped (with rather undue haste) one honour after another on him. He received the Freedom of the City of Berlin, and Kaiser Wilhelm personally presented the Grand Cross of the Red Eagle to him. Could great men such as Robert Koch make a mistake? Well, unfortunately, yes! It was not just a mistake; it was a fiasco. Tuberculin was administered to thousands of individuals with tuberculosis over the next year, and in many patients, the cure worsened the disease. Koch was now denounced for making baseless claims and for not revealing the nature of his 'remedy'. In 1891, Koch published a paper stating that his 'cure' was the glycerine extract of the tubercle bacilli. A few scorned him for a revelation made too late. Yet in years to come, tuberculin did have and continues to have a diagnostic use. An intradermal injection would often produce a strong reaction if the patient in the past or present had been infected by the tubercle bacillus.

Notwithstanding Koch's debacle on the use of tuberculin, the glory of his early discoveries remained undimmed, and in 1905, he was awarded the Nobel Prize. He was revered but perhaps not as universally respected as Pasteur. Like Pasteur he gathered around him a wealth of talented scientists who contributed significantly to the science he had pioneered.

* * *

An army of microbiologists, physicians and surgeons who waged a war against infectious diseases followed these four pioneers. It was not enough to identify specific micro-organisms, each causing a specific disease. It was important to successfully combat these infections. Many infections were prevented, as Pasteur had predicted, following the use of a specific vaccine against a specific disease. This was not however enough. Drugs needed to be discovered to help the fight against infection. Sulphonamides were the first important group of drugs that were shown to combat gram-positive infections. The close association between industry, science, technology and medicine governed mankind's fight against infection in the late nineteenth and early twentieth centuries. Pharmaceutical companies could provide a mass supply of sulphonamides, and the pharmaceutical industry flourished. Even so, the interests of the industry were not necessarily parallel to the interests of medical science. The former's chief interest was profit; the latter's directed solely into getting to know the unknown. Ethical problems and clashes were bound to arise and continue to do so in present times.

A great step in the fight against infection was the discovery of the antibiotic penicillin in 1928 by Alexander Fleming, a Scottish microbiologist at St Mary's Hospital. This opened the door to the discovery of numerous other antibiotics. We live in an antibiotic era, using increasingly powerful antibiotics that until recently acted against a wide range of micro-organisms. As recently as the 1980s, specialists in infectious diseases exulted that infections had by and large been conquered and that very soon infectious diseases could be considered a blemish and an accident of the past. These wise men were grievously mistaken.

Infections not only continue to exist, they flourish. It is not sufficiently realized that there is an ecological balance between Man and the invisible world of micro-organisms. A marked disturbance of this ecological balance is fraught with great risk to Man. We seem to have forgotten that Man has evolved over millions of years through selective mutation enabling the survival of the fittest. The overuse and misuse of broad-spectrum antibiotics has led to the mutation of organisms so that they are now resistant to the very antibiotics to which they were earlier susceptible. It is under the intense pressure of antibiotics that these organisms mutate and acquire resistance; they are indeed forced to mutate if they are to survive—again a question of survival of the fittest.

We may soon be left with a world of marauding drug-resistant organisms causing untreatable infections. The benefits to mankind initiated by the pioneering work of the great scientists of the nineteenth and twentieth centuries may well be lost. Medicine may then be forced to once again go back to the beginning.

3

Medical Ethics

Only a good man can be great physician.

—HERMANN NOTHNAGEL

Medical ethics is one branch of general ethics, and it would be wrong to divorce the ethics of medicine from the ethics of everyday life. Professor Dunstan gives a succinct but good definition of medical ethics—'obligations of a moral nature which govern the practice of medicine'. It is important to dwell briefly on this definition—on the implications of the term 'obligations of a moral nature' and as to what constitutes 'the practice of medicine'.

'Moral' and 'ethical' are for all practical purposes interchangeable words. The term 'moral' raises the practical issues of good and evil or right and wrong and of one's obligation as a physician to choose the good or right course. This is not always easy or apparent because one moral obligation right by itself may conflict with another different but equally righteous moral obligation in a given circumstance. Ethical principles are often rooted in religious, philosophical, or sociocultural traditions. These may vary in different societies and different civilizations. It can become increasingly difficult to establish an agreed ethical code in a number of situations when there is a wide variation in the moral base. Even so, the absolute values of good and evil, right and wrong, and the belief in the sanctity of human life are remarkably similar in all civilized societies. The practice of medicine is in equal measure an art and a science. It is the art and the philosophical aspects of medicine far more than its science that help the physician see through ethical or moral quandaries faced in clinical practice.

The history of medical ethics stretches back to antiquity. The Code of Hammurabi (1500 BCE), the King of Babylon, stresses that the physician's duty is to do good to the patient. The Hippocratic Oath (fifth century BCE), and the *Charaka Samhita* and *Sushruta Samhita* (second century CE) are more specific on various ethical issues. The first code of medical ethics, *Formula Comitis Archiatrorum*, was published in the fifth century CE during the reign of the Ostrogothic king Theodoric the Great. In the Medieval era, Islamic physicians made a significant contribution to ethics in relation to medicine. Prominent among these physicians were Ishaq ibn Ali al-Ruhawi, who wrote the first book dedicated to medical ethics; Avicenna, who wrote the *Canon of Medicine*; and Abū Bakr Muhammad ibn Zakariyyā al-Rāzī (known as 'Rhazes' in the West), one of the best known physicians of that age. Contributions to medical ethics also came from Jewish physicians and thinkers, such as Maimonides; from Roman Catholic scholastic thinkers, such as Thomas Aquinas; and from the case-oriented analysis (casuistry) of Catholic moral theology.

In the eighteenth and nineteenth centuries, a more detailed discourse on ethics ensued. Thomas Percival, a physician and author, crafted a code of medical ethics in 1794 and wrote an expanded version in 1804. The twentieth century (1960s and 1970s) saw a more liberal approach to the application of ethical principles in medicine. Medical ethics underwent a dramatic change and was refigured into bioethics.

From antiquity to the present, medicine is as much a moral enterprise as one based on its art and science. Tom Beauchamp and James Childress in their textbook *Principles of Biomedical Ethics* recognize four basic moral principles that constitute the foundation of modern medical ethics. These basic accepted moral obligations in a doctor–patient relationship are Beneficence, and its companion-in-arms, Non-maleficence, Autonomy and Justice. It is a judicious balance between these obligations that determines ethical decisions in a given clinical situation.

Beneficence and Non-maleficence

This is the core principle in medical ethics. It means doing good to the patient and acting in the best interests of the patient (*salus aegroti suprema lex*). A necessary requisite to confer beneficence is the expertise and skill of the practising physician in a given situation. If the expertise is lacking, it becomes incumbent to enlist the help of a colleague who possesses the expertise. In my opinion, beneficence includes far more than mere medical expertise and skill. It should also include human qualities—qualities that have been pushed into the background in modern times by the hubris of advancing science and technology. The essence of these human qualities is humanity or humanism. Humanity can be defined as the quality that enables a physician to truly care for his patient, to help cure him or relieve him of his suffering. The practice of humanism or humanity belongs to the domain of the art of medicine. The art of medicine is difficult to describe; it cannot be quantified as can its science. It consists of qualities of the heart and mind, which enable the physician to truly empathize with the patient; it cements the doctor–patient relationship, which lies at the heart of clinical medicine and helps in healing. Unfortunately, as I see it, it is a forgotten art. It may well become a lost art; this will indeed be a detriment to the practice of medicine.

Non-maleficence is the counterpart of beneficence. It means that it is the physician's duty to ensure that he does no harm to the patient as illustrated by the principle *primum non nocere*—first of all, do no harm. This principle is as much or even more important than beneficence—doing good to the patient. But, at times, harm comes to the patient in spite of the best efforts of the physician. An illness may necessitate a form of treatment that is effective and could result in a cure but could also be associated with side effects that could harm or even kill the patient—what is termed 'a double effect'. The ethical principle is to come to a decision on an investigation, procedure, or form of treatment only after carefully weighing the good that can accrue versus the possible harm that can follow. The most carefully made decision may, however, still go awry and may do more harm than good.

Autonomy

Patient autonomy signifies the right of the patient to determine whether he or she accepts or rejects a form of treatment the doctor advises. The patient also has the right to agree or disagree to any diagnostic or interventional tests deemed necessary by his physician. Autonomy is meaningful only if the exact situation has been explained to and comprehended by the patient, with regard to the treatment advised or to relevant diagnostic tests the physician believes are for the patient's own good.

The principle of respect for patient autonomy has led to the development of patient-centred medicine. It has been used to criticize medical paternalism and has led to changing attitudes towards the doctor–patient relationship. Respect for patient autonomy has led to providing patients with full information and to the concept of informed consent. It is also an important ground for the preservation of patient confidentiality.

It is important to realize that autonomous decisions made by a patient when contrary to the advice of the treating doctor should be rational, in accord with the patient's interests, and based on critical reflection. If the patient's choice is not based on critical reflection, many would consider it as non-autonomous. Hence, respecting a person's autonomy is not necessarily the same as respecting his choice. There are perhaps a number of physicians in the West, particularly in the United States, who would disagree with this statement.

In clinical practice, ethical quandaries arise when there is a conflict between beneficence (doing good to the patient and acting in his best interests) and autonomy (respecting the patient's wishes). It is the proper interpretation of the balance between beneficence and autonomy that governs decision-making in medicine. If a conflict between these two principles does arise in emergency or critical care medicine, the physician must lean towards the principle of beneficence and take management decisions that he or she truly believes are in the best interests of the patient. Let me cite a few examples in relation to critically ill patients to illustrate this point.

Mr B, a thirty-year-old man, married with two children, was admitted to the ICU with severe pneumonia. He was cyanosed with an oxygen saturation of < 70%, was gasping with a shallow respiratory rate of 50/min, had a tachycardia of 160/min, and was markedly hypotensive. He was dying of hypoxia but refused intubation with mechanical ventilatory support. He refused 'to have a machine fixed on him'; he cited his right to refuse treatment, and he was prepared to sign a statement to this effect. He claimed he would rather accept death than be ventilated. We did not waste time—we intubated him against his wish, ventilated him, and gave him the necessary antibiotics and other supportive treatment. He recovered completely after a stormy illness. On recovery he was grateful for what we had done, sorry for having been so difficult, and distributed chocolates to the staff of the ICU!

Let me give just one more example in acute medicine where there is a conflict between beneficence and autonomy. A young lady doctor was brought into the ICU, deeply comatose, with a note saying that she had poisoned herself on purpose, and it was her rightful wish that if by chance she was brought to hospital she should not be resuscitated. She was indeed close to death. Her suicide note was disregarded, and all attempts were made to resuscitate her and bring her back to life. We succeeded in doing so. Again the patient was happy to be alive and very grateful that we had ignored her note and set her right.

It is important to realise that there are many factors that distort, prejudice, or interfere with autonomous decisions in critically ill patients. These include fear, anxiety, depression, panic, and antagonism to hospitals, to machines, and to the medical profession in general. Critical thinking is often absent in acute critically ill patients. Respecting a patient's autonomy in such instances is not necessarily the same as respecting the patient's choice or wish.

The situation is different in chronic problems. For example, one must respect the autonomous decision of a patient to refuse radiation or chemotherapy after he or she has been clearly informed and has understood the implications of such a decision. This respect holds for any informed decision a patient may make in different clinical situations.

However, respect for a patient's autonomy may be problematic in certain situations:

A. When to do so would counter the principle of bene-ficence and results in harm to the patient.

As mentioned earlier, the working ethical principle in critically ill patients when faced with a life-threatening reversible situation is that beneficence prevails over patient autonomy.

There are, however, numerous other situations where respecting patient autonomy may almost certainly harm the patient thereby negating the core principle of beneficence. Would it be ethical for a physician under such circumstances to persuade the patient that it is in his own best interests to change an autonomous decision? I think it is perfectly ethical to do so in our existing sociocultural milieu. This approach would be anathema to a number of practicing physicians in the West, particularly in the United States, where patient autonomy is sacrosanct even under emergency conditions. A change in the patient's attitude towards an autonomous decision that is contrary to beneficence can often (though not always) come about if there is a strong bond between the physician and the patient—a close doctor–patient relationship. If the patient has faith in the physician and is convinced that the physician truly cares and has the patient's interest close to his heart and if the patient finally realizes that the physician is better aware and knowledgeable about the solution to his predicament, the patient may then ultimately decide to be guided by what the physician sincerely believes is right for him and in his best interests. This can only happen if the physician, in addition to his skills, is humane in his approach to medicine. It can only happen if he practises the art of medicine together with its science. I call this approach to the conflict between beneficence and autonomy as 'soft paternalism'. When practised judiciously, it enhances and reinforces the basic principle of beneficence.

How does a physician react if persuasion or soft paternalism fails to change a patient's autonomous decision in the previously mentioned situation? The physician then abides by the patient's autonomous decision. It is no surprise if the patient changes his decision on his own when he becomes even more ill (often hopelessly so) and requests the physician to act as he thinks fit. However, if an autonomous decision in a given situation goes strongly against the grain of the conscience or the moral obligation of the physician, he has the right to be relieved of his responsibility.

I need to cite one more example to illustrate this issue.

A patient known to me for several years had diverticulitis. She had repeated exacerbations of this disease. When advised surgery with lengthy explanations as to its possible complications, she exercised her right to persist with medical treatment. Then on one occasion she had a severe attack leading to a perforation of the colon and a localized abscess abutting on the bladder. She developed sepsis; she required surgery, which she emphatically and persistently refused. Realizing the danger she was in, I explained that though I had respected her earlier decisions against surgery, this was different. She needed guidance and needed to follow this guidance for her own good. If she had faith in me and if she admitted that I was deeply concerned over her predicament, she should eschew her decision and be guided by what I sincerely felt was best for her. All this was said not just in the few words stated above, but by lengthy talks and discussions that finally made her change her mind. It was not forcing a decision on her but guiding her to accept a decision that was in her own interest. The results were of course gratifying, both for the patient and me.

B. When to do so would harm others. The conflict between respecting autonomy vis-à-vis harm to the patient
and to others also arises with respect to confidentiality.
I shall briefly touch upon this later.
C. When the patient lacks the capacity to make a decision.
In such a situation, how does one respect the patient's
autonomy?

I need to give an example to illustrate this aspect at
length.

Mr B, a wealthy businessman, loves art and is
passionately fond of music. His father and uncle
both suffered from Alzheimer's disease. Because he is
occasionally forgetful, he felt he could suffer likewise.
He was otherwise perfectly mentally competent and
capable but expressed a wish that if he did develop
Alzheimer's and was mentally incapacitated he should
be allowed to die if he suffered any physical illness.
He did develop full-blown Alzheimer's over the next
four years, but it was a happy Alzheimer's! He can
recognize his wife but no one else. He is looked after
perfectly in his own home. He listens to music and
watches TV, admires his art collection, loves his drink
and his food, and is always smiling and laughs easily.
He developed an acute urinary tract infection resulting
in severe sepsis. His blood culture was positive for
gram-negative infection. If treated with appropriate
antibiotics he would recover, else he would almost
certainly die.

Does one respect his autonomy by not giving
antibiotics and allow him to die? This is consistent with
his wishes expressed when he was mentally competent.
Again, we have autonomy versus beneficence. There
are certain concerns that should prevent us from
allowing autonomy to prevail. Could Mr B have
known when he expressed his view to be allowed to

die what his current situation would be? Did he take into account the possibility that he would be enjoying life even though he developed Alzheimer's? At what stage of Alzheimer's would he want to be allowed to die? Would he have refused an antibiotic if with Alzheimer's he was happy and content with life? Also is it possible that he might have changed his mind before losing his mental capacity? Finally, it is difficult for a patient who is healthy with a sound mind to imagine the extent of disability that would accrue in his own individual case. There are some who would respect the patient's autonomy and allow him to die. I would disagree, for I feel that he may not have understood and taken into consideration the relevant issues stated here and that his expressed wish was, therefore, not truly autonomous. I would tilt towards beneficence, treat him with antibiotics so that he lives, continues to remain smiling and happy, and continues to enjoy the simple pleasures of life. This would be beneficent and in his best interests.

In most situations, where a patient is not mentally capable, there will not be sufficient information about his views and values (when mentally competent) to make a decision as to how to act and what to do based mainly on the principle of autonomy. It is best in these situations to practise beneficence and treat such patients in their best interest.

Best Interests

It has been repeatedly mentioned that beneficence means doing good to the patient by acting in his best interests. How does one judge a patient's best interest? A physician's concept of 'best interest' may differ from that of the patient. Also best interests may differ in different societies depending on religious, philosophical and sociocultural influences. Let me first briefly state what best interests mean to most practicing physicians in the West.

The philosophical discussion on best interests in the West is directed towards the concept of well-being. There are three aspects or approaches to well-being. These are briefly mentioned with reference to the case history of Mr B.

1. The first approach considers 'hedonistic theories of well-being', which hold that well-being as a mental state in which happiness is the intrinsic good and unhappiness or pain, the intrinsic bad. In this approach, Mr B with Alzheimer's disease is happy and it would be in his best interest, as already stated, to treat his infection.

2. The second approach considers 'desire-fulfilling theories of well-being', which hold that well-being consists of fulfilment of those desires pertaining to life as a whole. The desire-fulfilling theories of well-being point to respecting autonomy, but they are not the same. In the case of Mr B, did he have any relevant desires at the time he was or was not to receive antibiotics for his urinary infection? He obviously did not have the mental capacity and therefore the autonomy to express his desire.

3. The third approach considers the 'objective list theories of well-being', which holds well-being to comprise a list of certain objective goods. Examples of items that may go on this kind of list include engaging in personal relationships, the development of one's abilities, and rational activity. But does it matter if instead of pursuing life goals, Mr B is content with the simple pleasures of life? Would one consider him better off dead or would one rather treat him and let him enjoy his simple pleasures?

In some Western countries and in the United States, the physician needs to consider each of these aspects pertaining to a patient's best interest before coming to a therapeutic decision. In our part of the world, where many families form a close-knit unit, the first approach, i.e., a mental state of happiness or even contentment, constitutes an acceptable state of well-being. The other two approaches are of less concern. In fact, a mental state considered neither happy nor unhappy is also acceptable by many who care for and love the patient.

Let us now consider a situation in a patient whose quality of life is very poor and where none of the three aspects of 'well-being' (a measure of the patient's 'best interests') apply. Let us do so with reference to the religious, philosophical and sociocultural traditions prevailing in our country. Here is a true to life example.

A lady in her mid-sixties had repeated transient ischaemic attacks (a reversible fall in the blood supply to a portion of the brain) resulting in transient aphasia (inability to speak) with a reversible loss of function (i.e., marked transient weakness) of the right side of the body. She expressed a wish to all those concerned that if she had a major stroke resulting in a permanent loss of speech and permanent loss of power of the right side of her body (complete irreversible hemiplegia) she should be allowed to die. Unfortunately, she did suffer a dreadful stroke. Though no heroic measures were carried out, she lived through the stroke; the quality of life, however, was now very poor. Her relatives—son, daughter and others—love her and are happy to have her and let her live as she is. Ethical dictates in our sociocultural milieu should prompt the physician to care for her in all respects and not take any measures that could possibly harm her. The relatives insist that though she should not be resuscitated if she had a heart attack, her nutrition must continue and antibiotics should be used to treat any intercurrent infection. Physicians seek guidelines in managing such a situation. I don't think guidelines can help in this and in so many similar conceivable situations. At present, the law in India would take up for the relatives if the physician refused to carry out their wish. Leaving aside the dictates of present-day law, I would care for her within the bounds of sense and sensibility, ensuing that 'care' does not amount to prolonging the act of dying.

CONSENT

The principle of autonomy requires the absolute necessity of informed consent. Valid consent requires three criteria—that the patient is thoroughly informed, that he is competent, and that the consent is voluntary (not enforced, there being no obvious or even subtle external pressure).

It is obviously important to ensure that the patient is competent to make a relevant decision. It should be noted that he or she may be competent to make one decision (e.g., taking a particular medication) but not competent to take another decision (e.g., to allow necessary surgery). If a patient refuses to accept treatment contrary to his best interest, it is important to assess the mental capacity of the patient to make this decision. If the mental capacity is sound, this decision is respected provided the implications of this decision have been very carefully and fully explained and understood. If, however, the patient lacks the capacity to consent or refuse treatment or a particular investigation, he should be generally treated on the principle of beneficence—that is, in his best interest.

How does one assess competence? This is of utmost importance and, at times, may be difficult. The first step is to identify all information pertaining to the decision. This includes the likely consequences of related but different decisions (e.g., different possible treatments or no treatment) and the possible effects both desirable and unwanted. It also involves the understanding of what would be involved in carrying out the decision.

The next step is to assess cognitive ability. Can the patient understand the information relevant to the decision? Can he retain this information? Can he weigh the pros and cons of the given information to enable him to make the decision? Can he effectively communicate this decision?

Finally, one must determine whether there are other factors besides cognitive impairment that can influence the patient's capacity to arrive at a decision. A delusional state or a manic or depressive illness may interfere with assessing information and arriving at a competent decision.

Making Decisions for People Who Lack Mental Competence

There are three approaches to this important problem:

1. Decision based on the patient's best interests: This has been briefly discussed earlier. If the patient's best interests are undetermined or uncertain, beneficence takes the lead.
2. Decisions based by proxy: An alternative approach is for a proxy to make decisions on behalf of the incompetent patient, if the patient has nominated a proxy when he or she was competent to do so. The proxy must act for the benefit of the patient. If a doctor opines that the proxy is refusing treatment that is highly beneficial, the doctor may need to seek a court ruling to overrule the proxy or may be asked to be relieved of his responsibility.
3. Decisions based on advance directives: Advance directives are directives made by individuals at a time when they are perfectly competent, elucidating how they should be treated in the future when they are ill and are incompetent to arrive at a decision relating to consent to treatment. Advanced directives extend

patient autonomy to situations when they are no longer competent. A fundamental concern in relation to advanced directives is that the individual may not be able to imagine the state of affairs of the situation at the time a decision needs to be made. Also an individual may have changed his mind in months or years after the advance directive has been made, and the physician is obviously unaware of this change. To the best of my knowledge, advance directives do not hold in a court of law as far as India is concerned.

Though beneficence, non-maleficence, autonomy, and the interaction between these are the basic ethical principles involved in clinical practice, we need to consider a number of other ethical aspects in a doctor–patient relationship. These have been dealt with below.

Justice

Justice consists of doing what is just and right and avoiding what is unjust and wrong. If, at times, this is not possible in its totality, then one does what appears to be most right and least wrong. Take the example of the tetanus ward that was set up at the J. J. Hospital way back in 1980. To start with, there were three ventilators among nine beds. There were times when nearly all nine patients needed ventilatory support. What does one do? As the most right and least wrong option, we would give ventilator support to the three patients who were most ill and most in need of support. But, then, what happens to the others who also needed support? In this case, we were fortunate in being able to transport them to an ICU of another hospital generous enough to treat them free of cost.

In the name of justice, physicians should be unquestionably involved in the ethics of resource distribution that provides, as far as possible, equitable care to the society in which they live and work. Unfortunately, in our part of the world, resource distribution concerning health is chiefly dealt with by the government in office and by politicians, with little regard to the priorities that need consideration in a developing country. As a body, the medical profession should pressurize and lobby health authorities for proper prioritization of health resources. For example, India needs large teaching municipal or government hospitals and institutions to be beacons of research, teaching, and subsidized medical care for the poor and needy. Large five-star private hospitals provide healthcare mainly for the affluent and not to the poor and needy. Justice also demands that the medical profession as a body should insist that rather than spending money on constructing large hospitals, the government should provide adequate nutrition, clean water, sanitation, housing, electricity, education— particularly female education—and vaccinations against communicable diseases. The importance for combating the scourge of tuberculosis, including multidrug-resistant tuber- culosis, has not been sufficiently understood. The medical profession on its own is unable to put the above in effective practice, but it must be unrelenting in pushing the health authorities to do so.

Communication

Communication is an ethical principle often partially or completely ignored in current times where physicians are seen to communicate more with machines than with patients under their care. It is not uncommon to witness during a round in a critical care unit the consultant and his team standing at the foot of the bed, studying charts, figures, or various CT or MRI images, and deciding what is to be done next, without even talking at length to the patient, leave aside examining him or her. The usual bedside ward rounds in many units are replaced by discussions on each patient by the unit concerned in a room where the data and progress of each patient is given by a computer. Again, there is very little communication between doctor and patient. To those of us who enjoyed and learnt medicine chiefly on ward rounds, listening and talking to patients and examining them, this is an unmitigated disaster.

Communication demands that a patient is thoroughly informed about his illness. He should be informed as to what is being done for him and also why, if necessary, what is *not* being done and the reason for this. Good communication makes a patient a close and cooperative ally, the doctor and the patient both joining hands to overcome a difficult problem. It promotes trust, and more importantly, faith in the treating doctor, and this unquestionably helps in healing.

It is of great importance to also communicate with relatives. This communication should be honest and complete, using simple language that enables them to comprehend what has happened, what is happening, and what can happen in the near future. Details of investigations, treatment given, and treatment proposed should also be discussed. This involves a lot of time, but a rapport between the patient's relatives and the treating physician is of vital concern; it also goes a long way to reduce litigation, if in spite of all efforts, the patient dies or is incapacitated.

When faced with difficult problems, physicians need to not only communicate closely with their patients and patients' relatives but also reflect and communicate with their own selves. How does one communicate with oneself? I do so by writing a lengthy summary every few days on what has happened to the patient, what was done, and by examining the *why* for all that has transpired. It also includes a projection of what to anticipate in the near future and steps to take to counter future events and complications. I have found that in a protracted critical illness communicating with oneself in the above manner lends clarity to thinking and improves judgement. It allows one to think on different lines when it is necessary to do so and helps one to understand the overall perspective of a protracted difficult illness. It is also a reasonable safeguard against possible litigation. To err is human, but to have detailed written notes shows that the physician has truly cared for his patient.

Charity

I guess there are many who would not consider charity to be an ethical principle. But in a poor country such as ours, it is an important feature of clinical practice. It is wrong not to see or to refuse surgery on a low-income patient because he or she cannot afford to pay the requisite medical fees. Medicine is not just a profession; it is a calling, a calling that in particular is charitable to the less privileged. As Sir Thomas Browne states in his book *Religio Medici*, 'No one should approach the temple of science with the soul of a money changer.'

Confidentiality

Confidentiality is a principle of medical ethics that is commonly applied to conversations during consultations between doctors and patients and is known as patient–physician privilege. The law grants protection to physicians from divulging their conversation with patients, even under oath in court.

Confidentiality with regard to patient records is important, except under extenuating circumstances where confidentiality could lead to harm to other individuals, the community, or the country.

Confidentiality is also challenged in patients suffering from sexually transmitted disease if they refuse to divulge the diagnosis to a spouse, as also in the termination of pregnancy in an underage patient without the knowledge of the patient's parents.

Traditionally, confidentiality was and is a non-negotiable tenet of medical practice. Currently, there is a more nuanced approach to this ethical principle, urging the need for a degree of flexibility in certain cases.

Honesty and Integrity

Honesty and integrity are features of everyday living that necessarily need to be incorporated in clinical practice. It is dishonest and unethical to accept presents, gifts, or favours from pharmaceutical companies. It is equally dishonest to promote their products through dishonest publications.

Respect for Human Rights

The great need for respect for human rights was realized following the dreadful experiments by the Nazis on prisoners of war and on those who they believed did not belong to the Aryan race. The Universal Declaration of Human Rights, adopted by the United Nations in 1948, was the first major document to define human rights. The Council of Europe adopted the European Convention on Human Rights in 1950. This convention applies the international human rights law to medical ethics. Furthermore, the Universal Declaration on Bioethics and Human Rights—adopted by UNESCO in 2005 to advance the application of international human rights law to biomedicine states, 'In applying and advancing scientific knowledge, medical practice and associated technologies, human vulnerability should be taken into account. Individuals and groups of special vulnerability should be protected and the personal integrity of such individuals respected'.

I have discussed the ethics involved in a doctor–patient relationship. It is equally important to explore the relationship between the medical profession and the practice of medicine in contemporary society, particularly in the Indian context. Does medicine offered to society at large conform to ethical norms? What are the drawbacks and failings observed in the current practice of contemporary medicine?

The stupendous advances in science and technology have changed the face of medicine. Medicine is capable of performing feats deemed incredible fifty to seventy years ago. This is an unalienable fact. Yet, paradoxically, there is today a deepening distrust, disillusionment, and even antagonism towards the current practice of medicine and the medical profession—a feeling also shared by many members of the medical profession. The paradox is doubly striking when we consider that around the middle of the last century, when science and technology hovered merely in the background and medicine had achieved little, the profession was held in the highest regard, and the doctor's image outshone that of any other profession. Today, when science and technology have pushed the frontiers of medicine far ahead, enabling medicine to achieve a great deal, the respect for the profession has plummeted, and the image of the physician is increasingly tarnished. To my mind, the reason for this paradox is that medicine to an extent has strayed from its path and lost sight of its goal. The mechanization of medicine and the hubris of its science and technology has submerged its art and robbed it of its raison d'être, its humanism. The doctor relates more to the machine than to the patient; the machine becomes the interface between the doctor and the patient. What is equally unfortunate is that the patient is made to relate more to the machine than to the doctor. This adversely affects the doctor–patient relationship, which is at the core of clinical medicine. By and large, collectively speaking, the medical profession does not relate to society as it should, and most thinking members of society realize this as an unfortunate aspect of current medical practice. The absence or near absence of humanism and humanity in contemporary medicine has left a lacuna in the practise of beneficence, a core principle in medical ethics.

The medical profession and its practitioners have rightly embraced science and technology. Both science and technology are essential features of modern medicine, forces that have given medicine a quantum leap into the twenty-first century. But there is more to medicine than science and technology. Technology cannot substitute for a carefully taken history or a meticulously performed physical examination. Technology will not help cement a doctor–patient relationship nor will it assuage the mental torment, fear and anxiety that may follow in the wake of an illness. I find to my utter dismay that the physician no longer ministers to a distinctive person but concerns himself with separate malfunctioning organs. Contemporary medicine often presents the tragicomic scene of a critically ill individual being looked after by a number of super-specialists, aided and abetted by the trappings of technology and science. Each specialist concentrates solely on his or her small exclusive field of expertise; the overall aspect of disease and of the patient as a human being suffering from disease is then easily lost.

To the mechanization of medicine is added the sin of commercialism. Money is a driving force in today's medicine. Its acquisition through the charging of unreasonable fees even from the poor goes against all basic tenets. The healing art is now more a business than a profession—a nefarious business that has become increasingly corrupt. What is more corrupt than the practice of doctors who on purpose refer unsuspecting vulnerable patients from one specialist to another for no reason other than profit? Or what is more corrupt than the immoral practice of commissions demanded by general practitioners from a specialist to whom a patient is referred? Corrupt practices such as these are common in the larger cities of India and perhaps occur in varying frequency and in various guises in other parts of the world.

One other major drawback of contemporary medicine is its crippling expense in relation to investigations, treatment, and the cost of hospitalization. This is partly because the physician of today has forgotten the art of medicine and remains deeply immersed in science. As mentioned, his rapport is with machines and not with patients; often it is technology, not clinical judgement, that dictates his course of action. Taking a detailed patient history is a forgotten art, as also is a meticulously detailed physical examination. Today's physicians forget to use their eyes, ears and hands, but remember numbers, equations and formulae. Expensive investigations and modes of treatment are ordered even when simple tests and simpler measures would easily suffice.

Institutionalized medicine has also contributed to malpractice. It is a matter of prestige that every hospital in less-developed countries of the world should be equipped with the latest in Western technology and science. Yet rapid advances in medicine render most machines obsolete within five to ten years. If an institute is to profit after spending a fortune on machines, it has to feed the machines and patients become the fodder for these machines. If an audit were to be carried out on the cost-effectiveness of modern-day investigations in medicine, the result might well be shocking.

Perhaps the underlying explanation for the decline in the ethics of contemporary medicine is a fall in the sense of values in most fields of human endeavour. A burning desire for material gain and wealth at any cost dominates life today. It is difficult for any profession to remain an island of high-mindedness and virtue when surrounded by a sea of filth and corruption. This is a possible explanation but certainly not an excuse. The answer is to reform and wipe out this canker from the heart of medicine.

Every relationship is a two-way affair. The attitudes of contemporary medicine require change, yet it must be remembered that it is society that has to an extent conditioned some of these attitudes. A great deal more is expected of medicine than it can offer. It is not sufficiently realized that there are limits to medicine—today and in the foreseeable future. Of all the diseases in the world, there are only a few which medicine can cure, though there are many that it can alleviate. When people experience this fact personally and also encounter the unseemly aspects of medicine with its escalating costs, it arouses disappointment, distrust and anger. The relation between the doctor and the patient and between the medical profession and society is inevitably poisoned. Litigation against the doctor for faults real or often imagined follows. The doctor learns inevitably to protect himself or herself by what is termed 'defensive medicine'—ordering unnecessary, expensive tests so as not to be held accountable if by chance he misses out on some rare medical condition. This raises the cost of healthcare. What is perhaps worse, the doctor often hesitates to interfere in a potentially salvageable life-threating situation, fearing that he would be held responsible if the patient succumbs. The ensuing encounter between the profession and society is detrimental to both.

In his book *Medical Nemesis: The Expropriation of Health* (1975), Ivan Illich, a professor of Sociology in Mexico, has written a rather scathing critique on contemporary medicine's relation to society. Illich contends that 'the medical establishment has become a major threat to health'. This is an overstatement, an exaggeration, far from the truth. Yet his contention that the medicalization of life has three major disadvantages raises serious ethical quandaries. His contention also carries a germ of truth and needs careful consideration.

The first disadvantage Illich mentions, which runs contrary to the ethical principle of non-maleficence, is the production of 'clinical iatrogenesis' ('*iatros*', in Greek, means 'the physician', genesis means 'to make'). Iatrogenic diseases in medicine are those produced by physicians either through treatment, procedures, or investigations, or are related to hospitals (i.e., iatrogenic or hospital-acquired infection). But then, iatrogenic disease is as old as medicine. It has been an inseparable companion of medicine since antiquity. The pharmacopeia up to the early twentieth century contained substances that must have done more harm than good. For example the frequent use of bloodletting and administration of noxious compounds must have harmed rather than healed, killed rather than cured. The only excuse for iatrogenesis in the earlier age is that medicine did not know it could inflict harm. But today we do know the potential iatrogenesis of medicine. Unfortunately, this awareness has not helped. Illich cites chapter and verse from reputed peer-reviewed journals in medicine to illustrate the epidemic of iatrogenesis related to contemporary medicine. Unquestionably, the more potent the drug, the more sophisticated the gadgetry, and the more invasive the procedures used in the diagnosis and management of disease, the greater the risk of harm to patients. Yet it will be impossible in the near future to separate the science of medicine from iatrogenesis. There is no drug worth its name that is free of side effects. Dreadful diseases often necessitate potent drugs (with inherent toxicity to the human system) and risky procedures. The management of patients with serious illnesses necessitates the taking of a balanced risk. While the use of contemporary medicine in such instances could result in relief or cure, it could also result in harm and even death. What determines the risk? It is not only the knowledge of science that determines this 'balanced risk', but also experience, wisdom and, above all, judgement—it involves in equal measure knowledge and the art that constitutes medicine even today.

Illich states that the second disadvantage of contemporary medicine is the production of 'social iatrogenesis', i.e., the creation of an environment that no longer has the ability to allow people in society to look after themselves. People are then hopelessly dependent on the medical system, and the medical system functions in a manner to ensure that this remains so. The medicalization of life would prompt people to consume medicines and seek hospitalization or medical treatment for inadequate reasons. An encouragement to take recourse to institutionalized medicine perpetuates the stranglehold of the medical profession and medical institutions over society. Broadly speaking, this would again represent an unhealthy and an unethical sequel to the practice of contemporary medicine. In my opinion, Illich's contention on social iatrogenesis, though thought-provoking, is exaggerated. Medicine and the society in which medicine is practised will always be interlinked. Both are dependent on each other, and their relationship needs to be carefully nurtured.

The third disadvantage of contemporary medicine is the encouragement of a 'cultural iatrogenesis' whereby institutionalized medicine has sapped the ability of people to face the reality of suffering in life and the inevitability of death. Modern medicine is geared to fight death to the bitter end, notwithstanding the frequent futility of doing so. It is now being increasingly accepted that medicine with its powerful technology and science should relieve all forms of suffering but should refrain from prolonging the act of dying. It is also being increasingly accepted that prolonging the act of dying is unethical and is in no way counter to morals or to the concept of the sanctity of life.

How, then, should contemporary medicine shape its values in order to improve the doctor–patient relationship as also the relation between the medical profession and society? The answer is difficult. Contemporary medicine needs to recapture the spirit of humanism and re-establish the special empathy in a doctor–patient relationship; empathy between the medical profession and society will inevitably follow. It is only then that medicine will win back its trust, restore its pristine image, and meet the universal respect and approval of man. Medicine also needs to stay away from the lure of money, raise its ethical standards, and place the welfare and care of patients above all else.

Euthanasia

No description of ethics in relation to modern-day medicine is complete without a short discussion on euthanasia. Euthanasia includes the following:

1. The intentional killing of patients who express a competent freely made wish to die because of the pain and suffering they experience.
2. Medically assisted suicide at the patient's insistence and wish.
3. Homicide following a surrogate decision on a crippled or handicapped patient with a poor or hopeless quality of life. In this case, the patient is not involved in the decision.

Advocates of euthanasia remarkably enough invoke the ethical principles of beneficence, stating that the act is morally justified because it is doing good to the patient and is in his or her best interest. In my opinion, this act is wrong, unjustifiable, and violates the sanctity of life as it is perpetrated with known intent to kill. Yet, it must be clearly understood that withholding or withdrawing treatment when it is certain that such treatment will be of no benefit and when death is inevitable does not constitute euthanasia (even though some prefer to call this passive euthanasia) because the intent is not to kill but to prevent prolongation of the act of dying. It must also be clearly understood that if a physician administers a drug to relieve pain or suffering (for example, administering morphine to relieve pain) and the patient succumbs because of the effect of the drug (the so-called 'double effect'), the physician is not culpable because the intent was to relieve and not to kill.

I gather from discussions with my colleagues in the West that a significant number of acutely ill patients who are about to die, as also patients with chronic but terminal diseases, express a desire to be killed or to be medically assisted in suicide. I find it amazing that in my long association of over fifty years with so many critically ill patients in their terminal state, there has not been a single individual who has persistently wished for euthanasia. There have been a few who have expressed a fleeting wish but talking to them and gently explaining measures to relieve their symptoms have led to a resigned and comparatively anguish-free acceptance of their destiny. Why is there this difference between the East and the West? I think it is basically related to sociocultural and religious differences. A patient's, and for that matter a physician's, attitude to suffering, pain, impending death, and death itself is conditioned by these sociocultural and religious factors. Most people in our part of the world and in the Far East believe that life cannot be divorced from pain and suffering, that we live in the midst of pain and suffering, and that each one in this world is apportioned one's share of pain and suffering. This is the law of Karma—a belief that one reaps in the present life what one has sown in previous lives and that one will reap in future existences what one sows in the present.

To die with dignity and to legalize euthanasia are slogans often linked together, as if one needs the latter to achieve the former. Legalizing euthanasia in our country, even in the most diluted form, could well open the floodgates to murder. Euthanasia, however, under strict clauses and safeguards, has already been legalized in the Netherlands, Columbia, Belgium, Luxembourg and perhaps in time to come, it may be similarly legalized in other Western countries as well. I am in no position to comment on the Western world, but for all the safeguards and guarantees against misuse that the Dutch, for example, have, is it not possible that a patient would want to end his suffering as a matter of a cult or even as a matter of duty that needs to be performed in time to come? Is it ever possible to quantify suffering? Is not suffering often a state of the mind? And can a state of the mind not be subject to changing social pressures and social mores? Can most doctors claim to have the knowledge, experience, and the Oslerian wisdom and perspective to be truly able to enlist themselves to the cause of euthanasia in a patient who states, 'I cannot bear the suffering I am going through'? These are pertinent questions that are difficult to answer. Finally, when one legalizes a solution to a problem like euthanasia, would the good that accrues clearly outbalance the evil or harm that could possibly result from this legal sanction? This again is a question that physicians all over the world should seriously consider.

Ethical Questions in Future Medicine

Future medicine will pose grave medical and ethical questions. The pace of development in the science of genetics in relation to reproduction and procreation has far outstripped the pace at which ethical questions are being resolved. Bioethics is an uncharted sea, and we need to map this sea if humanity is not to be wrecked on its shoals and reefs. The future will need to ensure the freedom of scientific research and yet safeguard human rights; it will need to strike a balance between science and humanity for the benefit of mankind and medicine.

At its General Conference on 11 November 1997, UNESCO discussed these issues and adopted the Universal Declaration on the Human Genome and Human Rights. The Declaration considered the explosion of genetic engineering techniques, their application to medicine and the fundamental rights of individuals to exercise choice. The Declaration states that freedom of research is freedom of thought and is necessary for the purpose of knowledge. It maintains that the application of research in genetics, biology and medicine concerning the human genome must be directed to the relief of suffering and improving the health of individuals and mankind.

The trends, however, are disturbing and I shall cite just a few examples for consideration.

There is an inclination in the West to identify genes responsible for 'good' physical attributes—blue eyes, the colour of the hair one desires, strength and intelligence. One or more of these genes could then be inserted into the fertilised ovum to produce the desired effect.

Inevitably, in the future there will be attempts to clone a human being even if there is a ban on these attempts. The moral philosophy that many scientists today consider worth following is that of Immanuel Kant, the nineteenth century philosopher and moralist. Kant considered each human being as an end and not a means to an end. Under this moral concept, human cloning stands condemned as unethical and undesirable. There is always the possibility of science being reduced to depravity and being used to clone a modern-day Frankenstein. Even otherwise, human clones will be the means to an end; they will not be valued as individuals in their own right but as 'copies' of those we respected or loved.

Genetic engineering is a subject of important research in scientifically advanced countries and in well-equipped research laboratories. It has already been practised in non-human species resulting in the production of a mixture of hybrid characteristics involving two different species. It is possible that in the future, perhaps the distant future, external genes (carrying attributes not observed in the human race) may be introduced into the human sperm or ovum in order to confer attributes that could change the human race. One must bear in mind the fact that the normal evolution of man over time, either through genetic drift or Darwinian selection, has progressed to the present state of Homo sapiens over millions of years. It may take many million more years for the further evolution of man through the above processes. Yet, the science of genetics can achieve this further evolution of man after perhaps a few hundred or thousands of years. It is anyone's guess how such a scientifically evolved state of man would appear or function. This may sound like science fiction, but what was thought to be science fiction some decades ago is now a reality. It is possible that the human race could be so changed that it would bear no resemblance to the present.

Strong enforceable ethical guidelines are needed to channel scientific research along lines that do not tamper with the structure of the human genome as it exists today. If these are not worked out and carefully supervised, then—to echo the words of Sir Winston Churchill—there remains the possibility that humanity 'will sink into the abyss of a new Dark Age made more sinister, and perhaps more protracted, by the lights of perverted science'.

4

War and Medicine

War is the only proper school of the surgeon.

—Hippocrates

Medicine is as old as man and must have come into being with the awakening of human consciousness. War almost certainly predates recorded history. War however has increased in intensity following the birth and growth of civilizations and the establishment of countries with demarcated borders. Ever since then, over the past four thousand years, wars have pockmarked the history of mankind.

War and medicine, though sharing a complex relationship, are striking contrasts. War is the supreme act of inhumanity perpetrated by man against his fellow men. In contrast, the guiding spirit, the raison d'être, of medicine is humanism and an abiding humanity. War stands for terror, suffering, destruction and death; medicine stands for the relief of suffering, caring, healing and life. Medicine, when treating a disease, does so by not only treating its symptoms and complications but also by determining and then eradicating the cause, whenever possible. However, in relation to war, medicine can never fulfil this cardinal precept. Medicine can and has evolved over time, through experience, innovation and research, to mitigate the wounds of war but it cannot eliminate war—a dreadful curse inflicted by mankind upon itself.

Military medicine stretches back to antiquity. From the Pelopponesian Wars (fifth century BCE) and the Gallic Wars (first century BCE) to the two World Wars of the twentieth century, and from then on to Korea, Vietnam, Iraq, Afghanistan and Syria, war has proved an exacting but efficient school for both surgeons and physicians. Hippocrates wrote, 'He who would become a surgeon should join an army and follow it'.

In ancient Greece, the Iliad described 147 wounds with an overall fatality of seventy-seven per cent. Wounds from arrowheads had the least mortality when compared to those inflicted by spears, javelins and sling shots. Wounds from heavy iron swords were always fatal. In this heroic age of Greece, every warrior was a physician. Homer mentions how these warrior-physicians were adept at removing arrowheads and javelin points from wounds, the use of pressure to stop bleeding, and the importance of cleaning and washing wounds and of bandages to protect them. These warrior-physicians were aware of the rough anatomy and function of the muscles, tendons, joints and bones of the human body. They observed how an arrow that pierced the heart would quiver with each heartbeat and how death occurred quickly from blood loss if the arrow was plucked from such a wound. They knew that wounds in the forehead and windpipe were the most dangerous of all, that a javelin thrust or an arrow piercing the breast could go through the lung, and that a thrust in the buttock could pierce both the rectum and the bladder.

Surgeons travelled with Julius Caesar's legions, and Augustus Caesar created a medical corps for each of his legions. After battle, the wounded were cared for. Roman surgeons tied ligatures, clamped vessels to control bleeding, poured vinegar into a wound as an antiseptic. Surgeons also accompanied William the Conqueror when his Norman army invaded Britain. These skills of yore were then forgotten or lost, for in the countless wars that followed in the intervening centuries, medicine played hardly any role in war. More often, unwittingly, it worsened suffering through methods that harmed rather than healed. Saving lives in early history and in the medieval era was never a priority. War was for destroying lives, not saving them. Wounded men were left where they fell and occasionally saved if camp-following wives found them. What little medical support was available was reserved for the nobles, knights and the high-born. One of the duties of a knight's squire was to carry dressings and ointments to treat his lord and master in battle. The ordinary soldier who fell wounded was left to rot and die. The hopelessly wounded were put out of their misery by having their throat slit or shot by those who survived. Those less seriously wounded were abandoned, and if they lived, had to find their own way home.

Gradually the importance of trying to save lives began to be realized both out of humanity and practicality. The practicality lay in getting the wounded well so that they could fight again. But the role of medicine in these early epochs was primitive and more often than not harmed rather than healed the wounded.

* * *

By the sixteenth century CE, the weaponry of war had replaced swords and spears with muskets firing deadly grapeshot and canons firing canon balls that could kill instantly or mutilate mercilessly. The carnage in war increased and was worsened not only by ineffective treatment but also by the wrong treatment of wounds that increased mortality. Then came on the scene one of the greats of surgery, a French barber-surgeon, Ambroise Paré.

Ambroise Paré was a young barber-surgeon who had joined the service of King Francis of France. Francis had great territorial ambitions and invaded Piedmont in Northern Italy. The wars that ensued led to great carnage and suffering. Paré (this was his first experience as the junior-most novice surgeon on the battlefield) showed that the usually prescribed custom of treating war wounds by cauterizing them with burning oil or a red-hot iron led to increased pain, morbidity and mortality. This was indeed a remarkable observation, an observation of a young barber-surgeon that saved many lives in future years. No longer were wounds, either in military or civilian practice, ever treated by cauterizing them.

Paré also noted that blood loss was the biggest killer in war. He devised the artery forceps, identified bleeding vessels, and clamped them to stop bleeding. He then tied the vessels with silk threads so that he could safely release the clamp. This might seem absurdly simple to today's surgeon, but in those times was an innovation and discovery that saved many lives.

During and following this period, the mutilation of limbs caused by war injuries necessitated prompt amputation of the injured limbs. Serious wounds were always infected; infection invariably led to gangrene, and gangrene of a limb meant certain death. The treatment of gangrene was amputation. Amputation carried a horrendous mortality from blood loss, infection and shock. Imagine the agony of the wounded soldier who literally had his limb hacked with a knife followed by the use of a saw that severed the bone—all this without anaesthesia. The amputation had to be done within a matter of minutes, the skill of the surgeon being equated with his speed, else death from shock caused by unbearable pain and irreplaceable blood loss resulted.

The next most important milestone in military medicine came during the Napoleonic Wars (*ca.* 1801–15). The carnage increased during these wars, with larger armies confronting each other and the use of concentrated deployment of heavy artillery. Wounded soldiers were left to die in the battlefield, as it would take a day or more to give them any medical aid. Many that were wounded beyond the hope of living were mercifully shot by those who had survived. Dominique Jean-Larrey, who was surgeon-in-chief of Napoleon's Grande Armée, noticed that Napoleon deployed his artillery from one place to another on the battlefield through fast horse-driven carriages whenever the occasion so demanded. He wondered if he could use this method to move casualties on the battlefield to a field hospital behind the battle lines for prompt medical aid. In his memoirs, Larrey wrote, 'When a limb is carried away by a [canon] ball, by the burst of a grenade, or a bomb, the most prompt amputation is necessary. The least delay endangers the life of the wounded'. He created what were called the 'flying ambulances'. These were horse-driven carriages that carried the wounded soldiers from the battlefield to waiting surgeons in a nearby field hospital. These carriages literally accompanied and followed soldiers advancing or retreating on the battlefield. Each flying ambulance was drawn by six horses and was equipped with medical officers and chests containing dressings for close to a thousand injuries. Napoleon supervised this innovation and gave every encouragement to Larrey.

The flying ambulances were indeed a positive and important milestone in the history of war and medicine. No longer were wounded men left to die on the battlefield, a practice that had been earlier observed over the millennia. In contrast to Napoleon, the Duke of Wellington who led the British army, was not overly perturbed by the suffering of his soldiers on the battlefield nor was he concerned with the importance and need of doctors. He was nevertheless impressed by the flying ambulances and ordered his men not to fire at them. The flying ambulances of Larrey were the precursors of the motorized ambulances that evacuated wounded soldiers offering prompt treatment in the two catastrophic world wars.

The credit of all advances in military medicine in the early nineteenth century belonged to the French. Larrey and his colleague surgeon-in-chief, Baron Pierre-François Percy, were always near the front line of the battlefield. Baron Percy formulated the lessons of war in relation to medicine in that epoch and authored the *Manuel du chirurgien-d'armée* (The army surgeon's manual). Larrey saw action in all of Napoleon campaigns—in sixty battles and four hundred skirmishes. In the Battle of Borodino, fought in 1812 on the frozen plains of Russia, Larrey performed 202 amputations over a continuous period of twenty-four hours without sleep or rest. Besides writing a biography of Ambroise Paré, he also wrote an account of his life as an army surgeon. Napoleon loved him and is supposed to have called him '*c'est l'homme le plus vertueux que j'ai connu*' (The most virtuous man I have ever known).

* * *

The mid-nineteenth century is believed to mark the advent of modern warfare. The industrial revolution, which fuelled the might of steam-powered factories, enabled war from this time onwards to be organized on an industrial scale. The first such war was the Crimean War followed by the American War of Independence and the American Civil War, culminating ultimately in the two great world wars of the twentieth century.

The Crimean War fought around the middle of the nineteenth century was a disaster of the first magnitude. Living conditions for the wounded British soldiers in Scutari (now Üsküdar, Turkey) were atrocious, care well-nigh non-existent. There were two redeeming features. The first was the work of Florence Nightingale who rectified the abysmal state of care and nursing, and who after her return to London organized nursing not only in the United Kingdom but also in different distant countries of the world. The other was the use of the anaesthetic agent chloroform, first used by Dr James Young Simpson in gynaecological practice in Edinburgh, Scotland. The almost unbearable agony caused to the wounded by even minor surgical procedures prior to the discovery of anaesthesia was at last ended.

The American War of Independence (1775–83) and American Civil War (1861–5) produced further advances in the surgical care of wounds involving different parts of the human anatomy. The seeds of specialized surgery, including orthopaedics, were sown during these wars and were further established during the two world wars.

The First World War (1914–18) and the Second World War (1939–45) were truly horrific. Technology and science had discovered more destructive weapons with the purpose of maiming and killing as many contestants as possible on either side—a soulless destruction that turned killing into an industrial process. Artillery shells causing high explosive blasts tore soldiers into pieces, rendered human beings unrecognizable, shearing off faces, shredding extremities, ripping open torsos, and burning bodies to cinder. Death stalked battlefields in many parts of the world. For those who survived the initial trauma and injury, death was not far behind, caused by bleeding, shock and infection. Physicians and surgeons faced a litany of medical challenges—where to start, how to stop bleeding, how to manage infection, and how to keep people from dying of shock. A triage system was put into place by France's medical authorities—a selection process to decide which patients should be operated upon immediately, which could wait for a few hours, and which were so hopelessly wounded so as to be untreatable and left to die.

Forty million people died in the First World War and seventy-two million died in the Second World War. The degree of human suffering was staggering. There arose a desperate need for new surgical techniques and new medical and other related technology, forcing medicine to innovate, invent, and adapt to counter the large volume of casualties and to treat wounds of varying nature, not encountered in previous conflicts.

The tragedy did not involve only soldiers on the battlefields but also civilians. Sophisticated weapons of destruction unleashed deadly bombs and missiles across great distances, at times more lethal to civilians than to combatants. In the Second World War, London suffered severe destruction from aerial bombs, as did Coventry in England. Berlin and Dresden were razed to the ground, as was Stalingrad in Russia. Six million civilians lost their lives in World War I. In the global conflict of the Second World War, thirty-five million civilians perished, including two hundred thousand in Hiroshima and Nagasaki from atomic bombs. Many who survived the atomic blasts died subsequently from the fatal effects of exposure to nuclear radiation. The Holocaust was a genocide that claimed the lives of six million Jews. The Second World War not only involved the land masses of Europe and Russia but also involved the land masses, cities and the jungles of Southeast Asia. The tentacles of war seemed to strangle the world, even involving the large Pacific and Atlantic oceans, where numerous sailors on either side met death from high explosives fired by naval guns, from being torpedoed by submarines, or from drowning consequent to destroyed ships.

Medicine tried as best as possible—in destroyed cities, in the jungles of Southeast Asia, and on the seas—to cope with these horrendous problems, but in many ways was overwhelmed. The emotional and psychological trauma of soldiers wounded, disabled and deformed, but yet alive, as also the emotional trauma of losing one's near and dear ones were difficult to overcome.

Wars in Korea, Vietnam, Iraq, Afghanistan, the Middle East, Africa and other parts of the world followed the world wars of the twentieth century. More death, quicker destruction and the use of even more deadly weaponry were met with better attempts by medicine to retrieve the wounded as quickly as possible, in order to offer early and better treatment, prompted by the advances in medical technology and science.

Yet, the misery of war did help to drive important medical advances that impacted the world at large. Before we deal with these we shall explore the close relationship between *war* and *disease*.

* * *

War, disease and famine are deadly comrades that have stalked the world again and again, bringing death and destruction to man even before the dawn of civilization. Throughout most of recorded history, it was disease—not arrows, swords, spears, bullets, cannon, bombs, or rockets—that was responsible for the maximum deaths. Smallpox, plague, cholera and tetanus were some of the many diseases that struck invading armies through history. What is more, soldiers infected with these diseases could spread many of these infections into newly conquered territories.

Let us take some reliable figures in relation to the American War of Independence and the two world wars. In the American War of Independence, seventy thousand colonials died in the war; for every one colonial who died of wounds, nine died of disease. Of the thirty-one thousand British casualties, only four thousand were killed in action. In the American Civil War, 304,370 union soldiers died of disease and were not casualties of battle. In World War I, a little over fifty-three thousand Americans were killed in action and over sixty-three thousand died from other causes. It is worth noting that the pandemic of influenza that started at the end of the First World War killed as many as fifty million people the world over—far more than the casualties caused by the war itself. The exception to this trend came with World War II, which resulted in more deaths from battle casualties (close to 292,000 Americans, for example) than from disease or other causes (113,000).

Battlefields are the breeding grounds of disease. Dreadful conditions, unhygienic surroundings, cramped living, often with rotting corpses as company, and contaminated water and food led to diarrhoea, dysentery and typhoid in the two world wars. Tetanus and gas gangrene due to infection of wounds by Clostridia present in soil were commonly observed deadly diseases. In the battlefields of Italy, Greece, and the tropical countries in the Asian and African continents, malaria was a killer disease. In winter, with troops huddled together in unchanged filthy clothes worn for days on end, typhus was frequent, often reaching epidemic proportions. The incidence of many of these diseases has fallen sharply in modern warfare because of preventive measures, but they still pose a problem in conflicts occurring in the African continent and other less-developed tropical countries.

The havoc wrought by typhus is instructive and illustrative. Typhus filtered into France from Spain in the sixteenth century and struck the French army encircling Naples (under the control of Spain). Half of the twenty-eight thousand French troops died within a month, and the siege collapsed. Emperor Charles V of Spain was left master of Italy.

In 1542, typhus killed thirty thousand Christian soldiers fighting the Ottomans. Four years later, it struck the Ottoman troops, thereby ending the Siege of Belgrade. In 1566, the emperor Maximilian II had so many typhus victims in his army that he was forced to make an armistice. His disbanded troops relayed the disease to Western Europe (including Spain and Portugal) and from there to the New World, where in conjunction with smallpox the disease ravaged Mexico and Peru.

It was typhus which was partly responsible for Napoleon's defeat in Russia. The disease set in after the fall of Smolensk. Napoleon reached Moscow to find the city abandoned and burning. During the next five weeks, the army suffered a major typhus epidemic. The unhygienic conditions were ideal for the spread of typhus—the freezing cold and huddled soldiers camping in the vast open plains of Russia encouraged infected lice to multiply within the filth and dust of clothes and unwashed bodies. By the time the retreat from Moscow started, thousands of soldiers had fallen sick, and those unfit to march were abandoned. Thirty thousand soldiers were abandoned and left to die in Vilna during the retreat. It was the bitter cold, starvation and typhus that decimated Napoleon's Grande Armée rather than the Russian army or the marauding Cossacks.

The interaction between war and medicine in Napoleon's Russian Campaign (1812) is further illustrated by a piece of historical research that has now come to light. Research has shown that Mikhail Kutuzov, the legendary Russian hero who commanded the Russian army and drove Napoleon's Grande Armée out of Russia, was shot in the head in a battle against the Turks in Crimea in 1774 and 1778. In that day and age, these wounds were always fatal. He was, however, operated upon, remarkably enough by a French surgeon, Jean Massot, who employed neurosurgical techniques that foreshadowed modern neurosurgery. Kutuzov lived; had he died of his head wounds, Napoleon would have surely been victorious in Russia. There is now one more twist to the story. The bullet wound Kutuzov sustained in 1774 had destroyed his frontal lobe. This had made him erratic in his behaviour, and it appeared that the injury impaired his ability to make decisions. Researchers are of the opinion that his brilliant strategy of avoiding battle (except for the Battle of Borodino) and avoiding direct confrontation with Napoleon could perhaps be related to the injury to his frontal lobe. Instead of giving battle, Kutuzov retreated with his army into the far interior of Russia. On reaching Moscow, Napoleon found the city burning and had to order a retreat. Freezing cold, lack of food and supplies, and an epidemic of typhus decimated the army during the retreat. Dr Mark C. Preul, Director of Neurosurgery Research at the Barrow Neurological Institute, who was involved in this research has said, 'It's a story of how medicine changed the course of civilization'.

Disease was used as a weapon in rare instances in the medieval era. Plague, also called the Black Death of 1347 to 1351, came from the East, probably originating in China. In 1346, it spread to the shores of the Black Sea where Italian merchants traded both with Central Asia and the Byzantine Empire. The Italian merchants fleeing from the savage tartars sought refuge within Caffa (now Feodosiya), a Genoese trading port in Crimea. Caffa was besieged for three years, during which time plague broke out among the Tartars. The Tartars catapulted dead, diseased, plague-infested bodies over the city walls causing an outbreak of plague among the Italian merchants. Those who survived and those still sick returned home by ship; they were the carriers of the deadly plague that erupted in Genoa. Merchant ships sailing from Caffa must have also carried plague-infested rats, contributing to the epidemic in Genoa and starting epidemics in other ports of call—notably Constantinople and the island of Sicily. From Genoa, the plague spread through Italy, and from Italy, it spread all over Europe, decimating the population. An act of war had indeed succeeded in causing the greatest and most devastatingly unsurpassed epidemic that the West had ever seen.

One other instance of the use of disease as a weapon is illustrated by the conquest of Peru by the Spanish conquistador Francisco Pizarro. When his ships crossed the Atlantic to the South American continent, a few of his soldiers and sailors were ill with smallpox. On purpose, he left these men on shore. The native population of Peru had never encountered smallpox, a deadly infectious disease, which they promptly contracted. Smallpox spread like wildfire in the native population, spreading terror and killing thousands. This diabolical act perpetrated on an innocent civilization went a long way in the Spanish conquest of Peru.

In modern times, there is the threat of the use of biological weapons as instruments of war. This has been tried with anthrax on a small scale, in the form of anthrax spores enclosed in letters and packages, leading to a few deaths in those who opened these packages. The danger of biological weapons unquestionably looms large in our world today as there are many virulent biological agents that could conceivably be used for murderous purposes.

It is not only the combatants on the battlefield who succumb to infectious diseases. War also creates conditions that allow these diseases to flourish in civilian populations. These conditions include the displacement of populations, overcrowded refugee camps, lack of hygiene, poor sanitation, lack of clean drinking water, and the frequent association of poor nutrition and even famine in war-torn countries. In addition, one encounters shattered economies and a collapse of health services, which were often inadequate to start with.

The beginning of the twenty-first century was marked by conflict in twenty-five countries, mostly in Sub-Saharan Africa. It is estimated that seventy per cent of deaths in these poor developing countries are due to endemic infectious diseases. Conflict creates conditions that have led to catastrophic epidemics of diarrhoea, dysentery, typhoid, cholera, pneumonia, malaria, relapsing fever, typhus and other infectious diseases. For obvious reasons, tuberculosis and HIV/AIDS become increasingly rife and difficult to control. Preventive measures and control programmes are poor or non-existent in war-torn areas, leading to an increase in vector-borne diseases such as malaria, trypanosomiasis (sleeping sickness), yellow fever and Lassa fever. Crude mortality rates sixty times higher than base-line values have been reached in wartime conditions, leading to large displacement of populations in conflict zones. The calamitous burden of death and disease affects not only non-displaced civilian populations living in war-torn countries but also as many as forty million refugees and internally displaced people worldwide.

The richer countries of the world have been slow to realize the importance of aid in every form to these poor war-devastated regions. Humanitarian aid is imperative not just for moral and ethical reasons. The globalization of the world and increased travel make it possible for disease in one region to spread not only to adjacent regions but also to distant countries of our world. The threat to world health security is on the rise. More than half the outbreaks of disease of international importance have currently originated in conflict zones, particularly within poor developing nations. Delay in detection, response and control of such epidemics poses a dangerous threat to countries all over the world.

It should also be remembered that countries afflicted by conflict are potential regions for the emergence of new diseases, such as Ebola in Uganda, or the resurgence of rare and old diseases. Poor countries lack the administrative structure, and the facilities, technology and trained medical workers to effectively counter and contain such outbreaks, which have the potential to spread to neighbouring and other countries. The tragedy in poor war-ravaged nations is perpetuated as the aid granted by rich Western countries fails to yield fruitful results. This is because of poor governance, anarchy, corruption, political instability, absence of health infrastructure, shattered economies, and because of the vulnerability of peace treaties between impoverished warring countries.

* * *

We need to explore one more relationship between war and medicine. Has war directly or indirectly spurred and led to the progress of medicine and medical research—progress that can be translated into helpful practice outside the theatre of war? If so, is war good for medicine? Many distinguished individuals feel that war has indeed spurred medical progress. A number of inventions, innovations and discoveries in medicine have been provoked by the hell and fury of war. Most of this progress was made by the exigencies created by the two world wars and was further refined through experience in Vietnam, Iraq, Afghanistan and Syria.

An obvious progress arising from war in earlier centuries was the treatment of wounds. As has already been mentioned, an important milestone initiated by Ambroise Paré was stopping the use of red hot cautery or of burning oil in the management of wounds. The invention of the artery forceps or clamp and of the ligature to stop bleeding, together with progressive improvement between the sixteenth and twentieth centuries in the technique of amputation of destroyed limbs were also major steps forward. As weapons of war over centuries became increasingly destructive, particularly following the use of artillery, explosives, motor shells and bombs, surgeons had to deal with different kinds of wounds in different parts of the human anatomy. Medicine innovated and adapted quickly using new surgical techniques to counter this problem.

Logistical organization, transport, and care of the wounded initiated by the flying ambulances of Larrey graduated in the two world wars to motorized transport of the wounded to first aid stations very close to the front, to field hospitals a short distance behind the front, and ultimately to well-equipped base hospitals.

In the wars in Iraq and Afghanistan, American and British troops were all equipped with tourniquets; if a fellow soldier lost an arm or leg they could promptly use the tourniquet to apply pressure and stop bleeding. A rescue helicopter carrying a doctor, nurse and two paramedics would fly out the wounded individual in double quick time to a well-equipped hospital. En route, the patient would be transfused with blood and also with extra plasma, which contains factors that help blood clotting. This protocol almost doubled survival rates. At the hospital, any patient suspected of internal injury would be given a full body scan. It is as if the full facilities of a well-equipped civil hospital had been transported to the battlefront.

The protocol of using increased plasma infusions for trauma patients has been introduced into civilian practice. Paramedics in ambulances are using military tourniquets, which can be applied with one hand, in increasing numbers to attend to civilian casualties.

Another important medical progress was the use of the portable ultrasound. The ultrasound was a military invention first used in World War II to detect cracks in armour. It was further refined jointly by the military and civilian doctors and is now used not only for scans but also to locate and anaesthetize individual nerves thereby relieving pain—an invariable accompaniment of wounds.

War has been a crucible of learning for emergency medicine and also for critical care medicine. The triage system first practised by the French in World War I has been modified and adapted to meet civilian casualties. Almost all over the world, emergency departments in hospitals engaged in civilian practice follow the triage system. The principles of management of shock and other emergencies, which were gained through experience on the battlefield and first aid stations close to the battlefields, have been accepted and further refined in civilian practice. The surgeon general of the US army comments thus—'most of the emergency medical response doctors in practice in the United States today evolved from medical experiences in the jungles of Southeast Asia in the late sixties'.

There has been a progressive improvement in anaesthetic technique and the use of anaesthetic agents starting from World War I right up to the present conflicts in Iraq and Afghanistan. Operations considered impossible were carried out with increasing success during and after World War I because of advances in anaesthesia. Similarly, the surgical techniques in dealing with various wounds encountered in civilian practice—whether they be gunshot wounds, stab wounds, crush injuries, or wounds resulting from natural disasters such as earthquakes, floods and tsunamis—have to a large extent evolved from experience on the battlefield.

Loss of blood has always been a prime cause of death on the battlefield. Progress in blood transfusion methods was largely due to the exigencies of war. Army doctors carried out blood transfusions since the seventeenth century. As a matter of historical interest, in the earlier centuries, attempts to replace blood loss in wounded soldiers was through anastomosis of the radial artery of an unwounded soldier to a vein of the wounded. Subsequently direct transfusion of blood was attempted on the battlefield and at first aid stations, occasionally with success but more often with disastrous results. This was not surprising as the knowledge of blood groups discovered by Karl Landsteiner dates back only to 1900. The importance of using matched blood was only then realized.

What revolutionized transfusion services was the addition of citrate to blood for its anticoagulant properties. It was then possible to conserve and transport blood. In 1914, Albert

Hustin, a Belgian doctor, used citrated blood for transfusion for the first time. Since blood could now be stored, effective devices were used to carry out transfusions at the front thereby increasing the survival rate of seriously wounded soldiers. World War II saw the evolution and organization of blood transfusion services enabling the storing of vast quantities of blood and the distribution of blood when and where it was needed. Blood banks came into being in civilian practice and were a boon not only to patients with injuries or wounds but also for all medical and surgical problems requiring blood.

Advances in surgery were not just limited to the care of wounds. The seeds of orthopaedic surgery as a specialty were planted during the two world wars. Neurosurgery, thoracic surgery, ophthalmic surgery and plastic surgery all received an impetus through practice in war. Many surgeons who specialized in these surgeries during war founded special departments in the fields of their expertise when they returned to civilian practice after the war. Perhaps the surgical branch that owes most to the atrocities of war is plastic surgery, and I shall use this as an example to illustrate how the horrors of war advanced the cause of reconstructive surgery.

* * *

The first grafts in reconstructive surgery were carried out in the First World War to help soldiers whose faces were mutilated during trench warfare—the men known in France as gueules cassées (broken faces). The main type of grafts were skin grafts and bone grafts. Osteoperiosteal grafts and Dufourmentel (tissue transfer) graft procedures were practised to repair disfigured faces. Harold Gillies was a hero of the First World War. He set up a plastic surgery unit in Aldershot, England. After the Battle of the Somme in 1916, he personally dealt with over two thousand soldiers with dreadful injuries.

Archibald McIndoe was another great plastic surgeon and was initially an assistant to Gillies. McIndoe learnt his art, craft and science from Gillies, replacing Gillies in 1936 as consultant to the Royal Air Force (RAF). The battle of Britain in 1940 brought over four thousand casualties with ghastly burns and injuries produced by ignited high-octane fuel. McIndoe felt that plastic surgery did not fulfil the basic objective in the treatment of such injuries, which required years and often dozens of operative procedures to rectify. He therefore coined the term 'reconstructive surgery'. McIndoe first used Gillies's pedicle graft—a large piece of skin from the donor site that remained attached to a stalk to ensure a blood supply till the new one established itself. For various reasons, he then switched to the cutting and use of free skin grafts, which took more easily and quickly. He was indeed an artistic surgeon endowed with great technical skill. These qualities together with his caring attitude towards his patients stamp him as a great surgeon.

In 1942, those who had been through McIndoe's ward decided to form a society club. They called themselves the 'Maxillonians', since the unit was officially a maxillofacial unit. A few months later, a badly burnt RAF pilot waiting for one of his innumerable reconstructive operations was heard to murmur, 'we are not fliers any more. We are nothing but a plastic surgeon's guinea pigs'. The society now named itself 'The Guinea Pig Club', and there were six hundred such guinea pigs belonging to sixteen different nationalities. McIndoe was voted president for life of the club, which continued to meet long after the Second World War ended.

The experience gained through war in reconstructive surgery was an immense boost to post-war surgical practice. It was also the start of aesthetic surgery practised not only on the face but also on various parts of the human anatomy.

Parallel to the progress in reconstructive surgery was the improvement in prosthetic devices for replacing an amputated limb or hand or foot. Prosthetic devices for facial disfigurement were also devised and refined over time.

* * *

Infections of wounds in war carried a high mortality. As mentioned earlier, gangrene often resulted, and the treatment for gangrene or impending gangrene when it involved a limb was amputation. War pushed researchers to find solutions to this pressing problem. M+B 693 and M+B 760 (discovered by the pharmaceutical company May and Baker) were sulphonamides that were pre-Second World War discoveries and were useful in the treatment of streptococcal throat infections, sore throats, pneumonia, gonorrhoea and other infections. Large quantities of these were required to meet the needs of the huge war casualties. The medical profession was put on a war footing so that vast supplies of these drugs were available by 1943. Winston Churchill was given M+B 693 as treatment for pneumonia, and in December 1943, he told the British nation—'This admirable M+B, from which I did not suffer any inconvenience, was used at the earliest moment, and after a week's fever the intruders were repulsed'.

Perhaps the greatest medical progress provided by the dreadful turmoil of World War II was the use of penicillin in the treatment of various infections, in particular infected wounds, severe burns and other diseases caused by organisms susceptible to this drug. The exigencies of war forced pharmaceutical companies, first in America and then in the United Kingdom, to mass-produce this drug. Penicillin was available for use by D-Day (6 June 1944), which marked the invasion of Normandy in France by the allied troops. The drug saved the lives of thousands of soldiers who sustained wounds and other infections. The Germans were unaware of this drug and did not have the benefit of this drug right up to the end of the war. Penicillin unquestionably contributed to Allied victory in World War II.

From time immemorial, sexually transmitted diseases (STDs) were an enormous problem in wartime. The Second World War saw an increasing epidemic of STDs, particularly in Italy. Penicillin was an effective cure against STDs and was responsible for successfully curbing this epidemic.

After the war, penicillin continued to be the wonder drug for several decades, bringing down the mortality and morbidity of several infections, including diphtheria, syphilis, anthrax, tetanus and many forms of sepsis. The discovery of penicillin also spurred the discovery of other antibiotics. Antibiotics against gram-negative infections (resistant to penicillin) were soon discovered, so that soldiers at war in Vietnam, Korea, Iraq, Afghanistan and Syria had a powerful array of drugs to counter infection and sepsis. The same advantage was also obviously enjoyed in civilian medical practice.

Besides the use of penicillin, one of the most important innovations of the Second World War was the development and use of the insecticide dichlorodiphenyltrichloroethane (DDT). The Allies first used DDT in the Winter of 1943–44 to control an epidemic of typhus among civilians in Naples. Its great success prompted the use of DDT in the control of malaria, which was responsible for both mortality and morbidity in several theatres of war where this disease was rampant. Spraying of DDT in areas endemic for malaria (Italy, Burma, Philippines, East Asia) together with the concerted use of antimalarial drugs and other antimalarial measures reduced the population of malaria-carrying mosquitoes and sharply reduced the incidence, morbidity and mortality of this disease. Allied offences in these areas would perhaps have been more protracted and less successful without DDT.

The intersection of war and medicine has generally been focused on the wounded soldier, the need to keep him alive and fit. Medicine has achieved this only to an extent through significant progress in the management of wounds, injuries, burns, bleeding, shock and sepsis. It is often unrecognized that more importantly, it is the treatment of the other infections and diseases that war brings in its trail, as also advances in preventive health measures, hygiene, sanitation, the provision of clean water, healthy processed food, use of insect repellents, insecticides and the enforcement of vaccination, that have contributed even more to the duration and well-being of a soldier's life. Wars have helped to stimulate a study of the natural history, prevention and management of infectious diseases. Prevention of infection was recognized as early as the American War of Independence and the Civil War. George Washington insisted that every soldier was vaccinated against smallpox realizing that an epidemic of smallpox could destroy the army.

War also brought in its trail significant psychosocial damage and disorders—the invisible wounds of war. Patients with psychosocial damage suffered depression, tremors, involuntary movements and behavioural disorders. These disorders were termed 'shell shock' or 'combat fatigue'. Shell shock was the precursor of today's post-traumatic stress disorder (PTSD). In the First World War, many of these soldiers, who in their disordered mental and physical state refused to fight, were called 'fakers', court marshalled, and even shot. The recognition of this disorder in later years has led to a more humane approach combined with psychotherapy in the management of this problem.

* * *

I concede that wars have unquestionably witnessed a number of advances in medicine. Even so, the increasing powerful technology of war aimed at death and destruction will inevitably and forever outpace all future progress in medicine and medical research aimed at countering these effects.

Let me quote Brain J. Ford who strongly felt that war assisted medical progress and research:

> If any good can be said to come of war, then the Second War must go on record as assisting and accelerating one of the greatest blessings that the twentieth century has conferred on Man—the huge advances in medical knowledge and surgical techniques. War, by producing so many and such appalling casualties, and by creating such widespread conditions in which disease can flourish, confronted the medical profession with an enormous challenge—and the doctors of the world rose to the challenge of the last war magnificently.

There are however some dissenting views and they need to be expressed and quoted:

1. Commenting on World War I, F. H. Garrison, in *An Introduction to the History of Medicine* (1929), said, 'The medical innovations and inventions of the war period seem clever, respectable, but not particularly brilliant'.
2. More recently, British sociologist Dr Roger Cooter wrote, 'For the most part, war has accelerated research into old medical problems of military importance, the bulk of which are highly specific to that context and of little value outside it'. Cooter further claims that civilian health needs have taken a back seat to the medical needs of the military.

I now, finally, feel the need to conclude this essay with a discussion on the interaction between history, war and medicine.

It has often been asked if progress in medicine and medical research accruing from and accelerated by the immense suffering, destruction and death caused by war is worth the while. It has been claimed that the same progress that was stimulated by war, particularly the Second World War, would have surely taken place in due course of time during peace. Perhaps the progress would have taken much longer to be realized, but it would have been free from the taint of death wielded by the sceptre of war.

A broader ethical or moral question is whether the good that emanates from evil is acceptable. The claim that discoveries and medical progress consequential to the calamitous Second World War could also have been made in reasonable time during peace is debatable. Out of a number of examples to refute this claim, I shall state two important ones. First, the use of penicillin accelerated by the exigencies of war; and second, the establishment and phenomenal advance of reconstructive surgery as a result of war.

A brief story of how penicillin was pushed into use because of the Second World War has been given in my earlier work, titled *The Forgotten Art of Healing and Other Essays*. It is evident that scientists Howard Florey and Ernst Chain might have given up their research on penicillin as they could obtain only an extremely small quantity of pure penicillin. It was only the outbreak of war that induced them to continue; yet, they could not even produce enough penicillin to conduct a clinical trial. British pharmaceutical companies refused to accede to Florey's request to produce the drug in bulk. It was only when Florey and Chain took their research to the United States of America that they could persuade (with the help of government pressure) pharmaceutical companies to manufacture the drug. Perhaps in peacetime, penicillin would not have seen the light of day for decades or may have never been put to practical use.

Similarly the advances in plastic and reconstructive surgery were because of ghastly injuries to the head and face of thousands of soldiers and air force pilots during the two world wars. The tremendous volume of casualties was instrumental in the advance of this specialty pioneered by Harold Gillies and his successor Archibald McIndoe. It could have taken many decades for this specialty to develop in peacetime, merely because of the comparative paucity of such injuries in civilian practice.

I shall now discuss the broader ethical or moral question, whether the good that emanates from evil is acceptable. The question of the acceptability of medical progress related to war would not even arise if war had become—or would in time become—extinct, and the world was forever bathed in peace and tranquillity. All medical progress and research would then have occurred during peaceful times. Unfortunately, war is a constant of history; it is intrinsically, inseparably woven in the history of Man.

The propensity to wage war seems to have been stitched into our human genome. To imagine a world without war is a utopian delusion that ridicules past and present history. In the *Lessons of History* (1968), Will and Ariel Durant quote that 'in the last 3,421 years of recorded history only 268 have seen no war'. From 1968 onwards to the present date, wars seem to be perpetually present with barely a few years free of war. Witness Korea, Vietnam, Iraq, Afghanistan, Syria—major conflagrations that have brought death and destruction. Witness the repeated skirmishes between Israel and Palestine, the genocides in Bosnia and Rwanda, and the conflicts between countries in Africa and between the warring tribes within this Dark Continent, which threaten to perpetuate this darkness.

History teaches us that we can neither wish nor will war away. I consider it to be a curse on humanity or a curse that humanity has inflicted upon itself. But many think differently. The Durants say: 'We have acknowledged war as at present the ultimate form of competition and natural selection of the human species. "*Polemos pater panton*" said Heracleitus; war, or competition, is the father of all things, the potent source of ideas, inventions, institutions and states.'

Yet, even when war can be justified to counter slavery or domination, it unleashes evil forces of destruction, disease and death.

How does medicine come into the picture? History, war and medicine are interlinked. War is evil; it generates evil forces. Medicine is the antithesis of war and stands counter to it. Just as war has evolved from the use of bows and arrows to the most sophisticated and destructive weaponry that is capable of causing unprecedented annihilation and death, so also has the art and science of medicine evolved from its roots of 'magic', to wondrous inventions and discoveries that have perhaps brought, as Samuel Johnson once said, 'the greatest benefit to mankind'.

Though overwhelmed by the calamity and destruction of the Second World War, medicine succeeded in mitigating to an extent, the suffering that ensued. This could only be because it learnt the lessons taught by war over several millennia—lessons that led to medical progress through innovation, invention and discovery. Progress in medicine with regard to the volume and changing nature of casualties on and off the battlefield is intrinsically and inseparably linked to the fury of war. Allegorically, it is the 'evil' of war against the 'good' of medicine. This is perhaps just one example of the duality that governs the world. Arnold Toynbee, one of the greatest historians of our age, after an in-depth study of history, religion and philosophy, believed that the best explanation of this world lies in the concept of duality—good and evil forces that contend one against the other. If, therefore, medical progress (good) is distilled from the burning cauldron of war (evil), philosophically, one would contend that no depth of evil can completely suppress good. We must, therefore, welcome this good from wherever it emanates for the sake of its goodness.

5

Tabiyat

*Medicine and Healing in India**

The groundwork of all happiness is health.

—Leigh Hunt

Let me begin by saying that though I have been requested
to speak on the traditional systems of medicine in India,
I do not practise Ayurveda—or any other form of traditional
Indian medicine. I practise allopathy, currently best known as
'biomedicine'. However, I have a passion for history in general,
as also for the history of medicine, which of course includes
the history of Ayurveda. I shall therefore speak mainly on

* This essay has been developed from a speech on the traditional
systems of medicine in India. It focuses on the history and evolution
of Ayurveda, while also briefly touching upon other prevalent
systems of medicine in India.

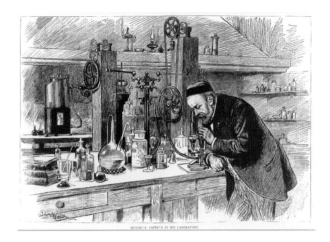

Figure 2.1 Portrait of Louis Pasteur in his laboratory using a microscope.

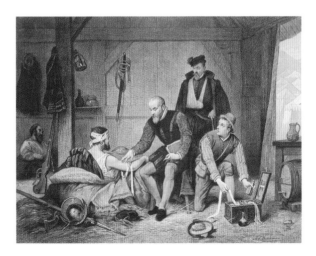

Figure 4.1 Ambroise Paré. Coloured line engraving by C. Manigaud after E. J. C. Hamman.

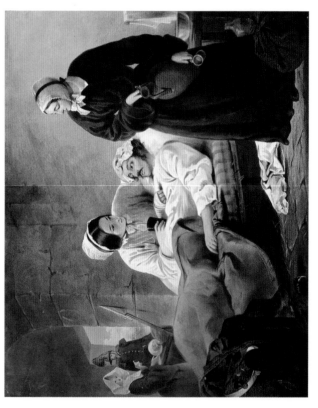

Figure 6.1 Florence Nightingale. Coloured lithograph.

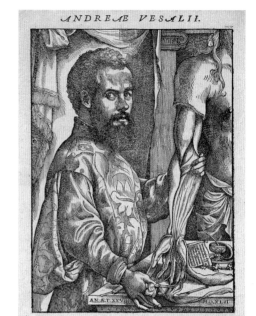

Figure 8.1 Portrait of Andreas Vesalius (1514–64), Flemish anatomist.

Engraving *ca.* 1600. Wellcome Library, London. Iconographic Collections Copyrighted work available under Creative Commons Attribution only licence CC BY 4.0 http://creativecommons.org/licenses/by/4.0/

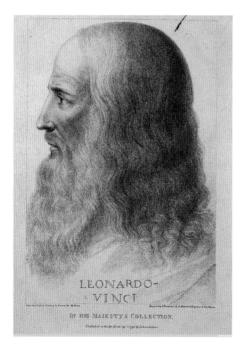

Figure 8.2 Leonardo da Vinci. Line engraving by F. Bartolozzi, 1795, after the sitter.

Wellcome Library, London. Copyrighted work available under Creative Commons Attribution only licence CC BY 4.0 http://creativecommons.org/licenses/by/4.0/

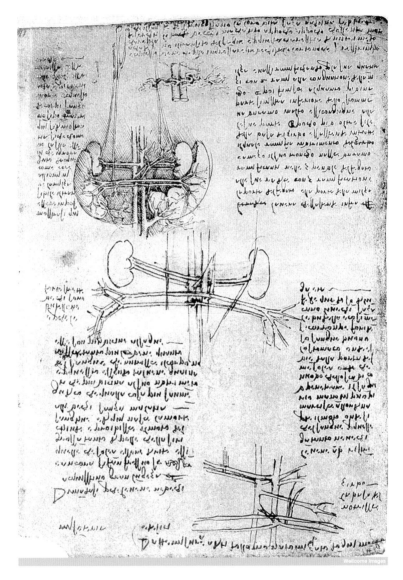

Figure 8.3 Studies of the abdominal blood vessels and arteriosclerosis. From: I manoscritti di Leonardo da Vinci By: T. Savachnikiff Published: R. E. Viarengo Torino 1901.

the history and evolution of Ayurveda, the most important traditional system of medicine in India, and touch briefly upon some other systems of medicine that prevail in this country.

The word '*tabiyat*', meaning 'health', is common to quite a few languages in India, including Gujarati, Hindi and Urdu. Though disease and its prevention and cure have been major concerns and preoccupations of humans since antiquity, the word 'health' is of comparatively recent use. 'Health' is derived from the old English word 'Hoelth'. In pre-Hippocratic times, health was considered to be a gift from the gods. If this gift was withheld or withdrawn, disease reared its ugly head. Hippocrates (*ca.* 460–377 BCE) was the first to refute this view and considered all diseases an affliction of the body, the mind, or both.

How should one define good health in present times? The WHO defines health as a 'state of complete physical, mental, and social well-being and not merely the absence of disease or infirmity'. But then, would an eighty-year-old man have the same sense of physical, mental and social well-being as one who is thirty years old? In a 2005 article, Professor Bircher takes this into consideration and defines health as 'a dynamic state of well-being characterized by a physical, mental and social potential, which satisfies the demands of a life commensurate with age, culture, and personal responsibility'. Today, health—besides being considered a state free of physical and mental disease or infirmity—is also considered to be a basic human right. True in theory, but far from reality in the poor developing countries of the world; disease, famine and malnutrition continue to stalk these unfortunate lands.

Unfortunately, many individuals fail to realize that good health is the most precious gift in life. It is only when 'tabiyat' is not good or is downright bad that alarm bells ring. It is chiefly then that medicine steps in.

I have often wondered, 'When did medicine indeed come into the world?' I believe medicine came into the world with the awakening of human consciousness. Modern historical research and the evidence of palaeontology and anthropology affirm that the roots of all medicine, in any and every country, lie in magic. The practitioner of magic medicine was the medicine man, variously called the sorcerer or the shaman. It was believed that evil spirits that caused disease entered the human body through various orifices and wreaked havoc either on the body, the mind, or on both. The shamans served to exorcise these spirits and remove them from afflicted patients through elaborate rituals, sometimes fair and sometimes foul; through the wearing of charms or bracelets; and through the use of hallucinogenic drugs.

Later, medicine came to be associated with religious practices presided over by priests. This was an important feature in the history of Egypt and other civilizations of antiquity. We thus have the practice of magic plus religion in medicine. This was followed by empiric medicine, and finally, scientific medicine. Even today, in spite of the advances of medical knowledge, medicine is well-nigh an equal measure of empiricism and science.

An Introduction to Traditional Indian Medical Systems

Ayurveda is the traditional Indian medical system par excellence. The origin of Ayurveda not only antedates the organization of India as a national state, but also extends beyond its present geographical boundaries. The history of Indian medicine undoubtedly involves large areas of land within South Asia.

A second great tradition of medicine, named 'Siddha', developed within South India. Though less well known outside India, it is of the same antiquity and authority as Ayurveda. Siddha was strongly influenced by tantric ideas and by alchemy. The use of heavy metals was extremely popular, and the Tamilians prized a substance termed '*muppu*' that was supposed to have remarkable power on the physical and spiritual aspects of man.

Rasa shastra is another ancient system of healing in India; it uses metal, especially mercury and gold, purified by using complex procedures. It is postulated that rasa shastra formulations, in association with yogic and tantric practices, confer special powers that counter the ageing process. Some rasa shastra medications were incorporated into Ayurveda and Siddha. The Sowa-Rigpa system practised in Tibet and the Himalayan region is an amalgam of Ayurveda and folk practices and carries with it a strong influence of Tibetan Buddhism.

Other medical systems originating outside India have filtered into the country and have been integrated into its culture, forming part of the Indian medical system. The earliest and perhaps the most important of these systems is Unani medicine. 'Unani' is derived from the word 'Ionian' and was the form of medicine practised in Greece five thousand years ago. It became a prominent system in the Middle East during the period of Arab supremacy and in the era of the caliphates. It was introduced in India by the Arabs in the Middle Ages and was the prevalent and preferred system of medicine during Moghul rule. Over centuries, it imbibed the features of Ayurveda. In fact, a fair mixing of these two systems is prevalent in the country today.

Other significant medical systems imported into India are homeopathy, naturopathy, acupuncture and acupressure. Yoga is an ancient endogenous system originating within the country. It is a system of knowledge steeped in philosophical and spiritual moorings but has been reinterpreted to focus on health-related aspects through meditative yogic practice. Finally, of considerable importance is the wide practise of folk medicine. This important subject is of special relevance in a poor country such as India. Folk medicine starts at home.

Parents or grandparents have a ready folk remedy for anyone in the family who has a cough or cold, rash, fever, aches and pains, or other bodily complaints. These remedies have been handed down for generations and are generally useful in offering symptomatic relief. If unrelieved, the patient in India may choose to step out of the house and visit a herbalist, or a hakim, or a palmist, or a hypnotist, or even someone who tells the patient his fortune and health by laying out a pack of cards. The patient may, perhaps, visit a god-man who will tell him or her what to do to propitiate the gods. He may visit the church, the temple or the mosque or plan a visit to pray at a dargah famous for its healing powers. If the patient has had an injury to a bone or a joint, he will visit a bone-setter, who at times is as good or better than an orthopaedic surgeon. In rural India, a delivery is often performed by the local *dai*, or midwife, who may be good but may also contribute significantly to maternal and foetal mortality. While, of course, the patient also has a choice of visiting an Ayurvedic or Unani physician, most of the practices just stated belong to folk medicine.

Folk medicine is of importance in India because it is the form of medicine practised in many rural districts, tribal areas and remote inaccessible villages. Remarkably, even in the large cities of India, there are a number of individuals who prefer to seek the help of folk medicine rather than other prevalent systems of medicine. It is also the form of medicine that antedates all other systems of medicine and is perhaps as old as Man. Folk medicine has no codified foundation or formulations and is instead based on a folk epistemology that gathers within its folds the diverse and often hidden aspects of folklore.

From pre-Vedic times, farmers, hunters and, in particular, those living in the foothills of the Himalayas have a remarkable knowledge gathered through years of experience, expertise and apprenticeship of the medical values of herbs, plants and roots. This knowledge has been passed on by oral traditions from one generation to the next through several centuries. Folk medicine must have significantly contributed to the codified, systemized texts of Ayurveda. A range of traditional folk therapies has been used to treat several diseases. Healing by using products obtained from animals also prevails. Folk medicine, additionally, includes the exorcising of evil spirits thought to cause disease through various ritualistic procedures. In fact, the practice of magic as a counter to disease is even today prevalent in a number of villages in India.

It is amazing that in some tribal and remote villages where the government has opened primary health centres, the tribals often prefer their own indigenous system of medicine, practised by herbalists, exorcists, snake charmers and the village dais. These are healers who have the people's faith and confidence. It will require a great deal of education before Ayurvedic medicine or Western medicine becomes acceptable to these people. If the old order is to change and yield place to the new, the new order must be so projected as to not violate their ancient faith. Till then, folk medicine will continue to provide some degree of service, particularly to those who have no geographic or financial access to the more scientific systems of medicine.

The ancient traditional systems of Indian medicine stated above, with their varied histories, have evolved over time. 'The development within these old traditions, the addition of new ones with the established ones, and their interaction and interrelation coupled with the weaving of medical thoughts with changing religious, social and cultural values have resulted in a rich, though complicated, tapestry of both the medical and social history of India.'

A Brief History of Ayurveda

The thrust of this essay is Ayurveda, which as mentioned earlier, is unquestionably the most important system practised within the country. Literally translated, Ayurveda means the knowledge (*veda* in Sanskrit) of long life or longevity (*ayur*). This classical and ancient system of medicine has been crystallized and systematically organized into a large corpus of writing in Sanskrit.

The first written evidence of Ayurveda was in the corpus of Sanskrit writings termed the *Charaka Samhita* (Compendium of Charaka) and *Sushruta Samhita* (Compendium of Sushruta). Charaka was a great physician and Sushruta a great surgeon in the days of yore, and these two manuscripts form the twin pillars of Ayurveda. There is another early text that has survived as a single manuscript—the *Bhela Samhita*.

The life and times of Charaka are uncertain. The name 'Charaka' appears as a great medical authority in the fifth century CE in the Bower manuscript discovered in Eastern Turkestan in Central Asia along the caravan route to China. Originally the manuscript was owned by the Buddhist monk Yashomitra, who lived in a monastery near the old Silk Route trading station of Kuga. The manuscript contained medical cum religious texts and was written by scribes in Sanskrit and Prakrit. After Yashomitra's death, the manuscript lay buried in a stupa dedicated to the monk. It lay undisturbed for a thousand years before it was unearthed by treasure hunters excavating near the ruined stupa. In 1980, Lieutenant Hamilton Bower was appointed by the British government to track down the murder of a Scottish gentleman Andrew Dalgliesh who was murdered by an Afghan tribesman while camping in the Karakoram Ranges. Bower was camping at Kuga at the edge of the Gobi desert when a man offered to sell him the old manuscript. Bower bought the manuscript for a pittance. The manuscript was forwarded to the president of the Asiatic Society of India, who sent it on to be deciphered, translated and edited by A. J. Hoernle, an expert in oriental languages in Kolkata. Hoernle retuned the manuscript to Bower, who later sold it to the Bodleian library in Oxford.

Further historical evidence dates Charaka to an earlier date. The French orientalist Sylvain Levy discovered the Chinese translation of an old Buddhist manuscript written in Sanskrit in the late fifth century CE. One of the chapters in this manuscript gives a description of the famous king, Kanishka. Kanishka, the manuscript states, had three companions and friends— his prime minister, Mathara; the famous physician, Charaka; and Asvaghosa Bodhisattva. The reign of Kanishka, though not absolutely certain, is considered by most historians to be around the second century CE. If written, scientific and historical evidence place Charaka in the first or second century CE, then how much further back in time do the roots of Ayurveda extend? When was the healing art and science born?

The origin of this ancient art and science is uncertain, controversial and clouded in mystery. A credible legend is that sometime between the second and third millennium BCE, the most enlightened sages, ascetics and teachers of India journeyed many miles to a remote Himalayan cave. They pooled their learning and experiences on the nature of human suffering and went on to discuss ways and means to heal and alleviate this suffering. Their discussion led to the birth of Ayurveda. The first great Ayurvedic teacher, Agnivesha, was a disciple of Atreya Punarvasu, a member of the original body of sages who founded the science. Agnivesha was instructed by the sage to commit all discussions at the conference to memory. Agnivesha taught his disciples, who, in turn, became gurus and taught their own disciples. This oral tradition continued through centuries till the body of accumulated knowledge was systemized into a written text.

Both the *Charaka Samhita* and *Sushruta Samhita* claim descent from the Vedas. This, however, should not be taken literally. The claim that they have been bequeathed by the gods might strongly serve to make them acceptable to those who learnt and practised Ayurveda and to those on whom the healing art was practised. Though the Vedas, and in particular the *Atharva Veda*, contain references to medicine, they bear no resemblance to the classical texts of Charaka and Sushruta. K. G. Zysk has provided evidence to suggest that Ayurveda as a system of medicine had its roots in the ascetic milieu of Buddhism that prevailed in India in the fifth and sixth centuries BCE. Written evidence in the earliest manuscripts preserved by the Buddhist monks in that period of history bears a close similarity to the system of medicine in the early texts of Charaka and Sushruta.

It is however possible that the birth of Ayurveda extends even further back into history, though concrete evidence to prove this might never be forthcoming. India, after all, is a land that even today is characterized by the oral tradition. It is in fact more than likely that the roots of Ayurveda and its early sproutings were passed on to numerous gurus and to their *chelas* (disciples) through word of mouth. The same analogy is present in Indian music, which was never notated and where the different *gharanas* (specialist schools or methods of classical music) in the country passed on their ragas and their variations through the gurus to their disciples. The disciples lived with the gurus all their lives, being treated like sons and daughters. It is conceivable that the little trickles in the ancient science of Ayurveda, gathered through oral traditions, became visible streams in the Buddhist period, finally joining together to culminate in the systemized medical treatises of Charaka and Sushruta.

Interestingly enough, in the text of the *Charaka Samhita*, the name Charaka occurs only in a statement at the end of the chapter, which gives the name and number of the chapter just completed. Charaka's name does not appear anywhere else in the texts, and neither is he termed the main author by his guru Atreya. Charaka probably revised and edited this work. The dates of Agnivesha and Atreya are lost in the midst of legend and time.

Finally, it needs to be maintained that though Ayurveda has no direct connection with the Vedas, the thoughts and philosophy introduced in the prevailing Vedic literature must have certainly served as a background that influenced Ayurvedic writings. This is proven by the fact that the knowledge of longevity, which Ayurveda stood for, was intertwined with the philosophy of life and living as enshrined in the Vedas.

The Philosophy of Ayurveda

The fundamental philosophical tenet of Ayurveda is that suffering is disease and contentment is health. Ayurveda recognized that suffering could be physical, mental and spiritual, and that good health necessitated a healthy body, a sound mind and a good soul. This philosophical concept transcended the medical texts, for it embodies a way of living based on the recognition of the interdependency of man with all forms of life. The spirit constitutes the intelligence of life; matter constitutes its energy. Both are manifestations of Brahman, or the ultimate reality, which constitutes the oneness of life. This concept stresses man's link with universal life; our health, even survival, are dependent on nature, and in not unduly disturbing the fragile ecological balance between nature and other living organisms.

Ayurveda enjoins that man's happiness lies in the ability to live in harmony with his own self. It is this holistic aspect in which man is just a microcosm, as also a holistic view of the physical and mental aspects of Man interacting with one another and with the outside world that make Ayurveda unique in the art and science of healing.

Basic Medical Tenets of Ayurveda

The first major doctrine of Ayurveda is that the body is governed by humours (dosha), body tissues and the relation between humours, body tissues and waste products. The three humours that regulate the body are semi-fluid in consistency and are wind (*vata*), choler (*pitta*) and phlegm (*kapha*). This theory is analogous to the Greek view, except that the latter includes a fourth humour, 'blood', and that wind is not included as a humour in Greek medicine.

Ayurveda also affirms that the body consists of a network of tubes transporting energizing fluids from one place to another. These tubes also carry the three humours, sensations, and even the 'mind'. Diseases arise when the flow of these humours is obstructed, retarded, or channelized in wrong directions. Great emphasis is placed on diet, and different qualities have been attributed to different foods. It is a remarkable fact that despite enunciating a great deal on ethical norms in life and on the style of living, Ayurveda unhesitatingly advocates the use of meat and alcohol as therapy in certain conditions and diseases.

A Brief Outline of the *Charaka Samhita*

The earliest of the Ayurvedic texts elaborates on anatomy, foetal development and the tri-dosha theory of the three humours that govern function and malfunction of the body. It describes the classification of diseases, aetiology, diagnosis, prognosis and treatment. Thus it discusses the cause, nature and management of different fevers, skin conditions, urinary problems, constipation, asthma, epilepsy, insanity, dropsy and several other pathologies. It deals with the science of rejuvenation and describes diseases of the eye, normal and abnormal deliveries, care of the newborn, and childhood diseases. The materia medica within the compendium consists chiefly of numerous vegetable products and also includes animal products and minerals. These are classified into several groups depending on the basis of action in the body. Treatment also includes methods to induce sweating, coughing, bloodletting; the use of leeches, enemas, and ointments and drugs from the vast array of plants, herbs, nuts and other sources that comprise the Ayurvedic pharmacopoeia.

The vast treatise gives the views of doctors specializing in different medical subjects; offers a code of ethics remarkably similar to the Hippocratic oath; describes the centres of learning and schools of philosophy that influenced medical theories; and provides information on medical botany, the classification of the plant and animal kingdoms, with special reference to the medicinal properties of the flesh of animals. It includes a description of customs, traditions, diet, exercise, and good and bad habits so as to be useful to the ordinary individual.

I do not practise or claim any in-depth knowledge of Ayurveda. In fact I do not subscribe to many of its beliefs. In particular, the theory of humours in the causation of disease is unacceptable to all who practise current biomedicine. There is no scientific proof whatsoever that the pathogenesis of disease is related to the imbalance of humours. Yet, there are undoubtedly aspects of Ayurvedic medicine that maintain health and counter disease. It is an incontrovertible fact that of more than a billion people in India, millions avail of Ayurvedic medicine and other traditional forms of medicine than Western biomedicine. What amazes me is that Charaka, writing his compendium over two thousand years ago, realized that the technical medical details of his compendium would evolve with time and that the history of medicine would be a chronicle of change. And indeed that has been so—Ayurvedic medicine has evolved over centuries like all other branches of medicine. It is equally amazing that Charaka believed and wrote that notwithstanding the change in technical aspects in years to come, the philosophical tenets underlying his medical treatise would remain unchanged for all time. Indeed the philosophical tenets of all medicine and of life and living are as sacrosanct now as they were over two thousand years ago and will continue to be so in the future history of man.

Other Notable Ayurvedic Texts

Let me briefly outline the Ayurvedic works that followed Charaka's compendium here. I have already mentioned the *Bhela Samhita* (of which only one manuscript survives). Another work of major importance was the *Ashtanga Hridaya Samhita* (Compendium of the Heart). Compiled in the early seventh century by Vāgbhata, it, along with the two older treatises by Charaka and Sushruta, forms the 'great threesome' in Ayurveda. The *Ashtanga Hridaya Samhita* synthesizes and summarizes medical knowledge, extracting the essence of medicine from previous works, and unifying and bringing order into its contents. This book by Vāgbhata is very popular and is found in many libraries both in North and South India, and is regarded as an important authoritative text on Ayurvedic education and practice.

Three later works have similar status to the great threesome and are called the 'lesser threesome'. These are the works of Madhava (700 CE), Sarngadhara (1300 CE) and Bhāvamisra (sixteenth century CE). All three works give a more current description of disease, and a number of copies are found in libraries all over India. Translation of passages of the above mentioned works can be found in Dominik Wujastyk's book *Roots of Ayurveda* (1998). In addition, there are numerous encyclopaedias and dictionaries containing Ayurvedic material. *History of Indian Medical Literature* (2002), a magnum opus written by G. Jan Meulenbeld, gives a comprehensive overview of Ayurvedic literature and is the most important book of Ayurveda to date.

Sushruta, the Surgeon of Antiquity

Sushruta, the great Ayurvedic surgeon, was the counterpart of Charaka, the physician. It is difficult to determine when Sushruta lived and wrote his manuscript. Evidence from various sources suggests that he lived around the second century BCE, at which time the core of his manuscript on surgery was formed. The manuscript was frequently revised and updated in the centuries before 500 CE. It is in this revised form that the world sees this famous manuscript today.

Sushruta of antiquity was a great surgeon, a great teacher and a renowned author. Like Hippocrates, he taught medicine at the bedside, gauged the aptitude of his students, and had the wisdom to teach only as much as his students could absorb and put into practice. He is believed to have innovated major surgical procedures and improved the general techniques of surgery. He also devised a variety of surgical instruments. He taught surgery to his students first on dummies and then on dead bodies. He was renowned chiefly for his operations on the removal of cataracts, lithotomy, and the removal of a dead foetus. He is believed to have devised abdominal operations; if true, this would indeed be a marvel for his day and age.

A description of Sushruta's many technical innovations is neither necessary nor possible in this essay; however, a fascinating innovation worth recording is the use of black ants for suturing. The technique involved bringing the edges of the wound very close together and then having black ants join the edges by biting through them with their mandibles. The ant's body was then twisted off, but the head remained, approximating the edges of the wound. Additionally, plastic surgery originated with Sushruta. Cutting off the nose was a common punishment practised on women for adultery and in males for a variety of offences. Plastic surgery to repair the nose or torn ear was innovated by this great surgeon.

Recent historical research suggests that after Sushruta, the practice of surgery by trained Ayurvedic surgeons declined and that surgery came to be practised by barber physicians as in the West. To what extent this is true is difficult to ascertain, nor is the reason easily discernible. The caste system had steadily grown in the first millennium CE, and this might have created taboos concerning close contact with those considered untouchables or those of a lower caste. Surgery, which involved close contact with patients, might have lost favour, and its practise by traditional Ayurveds may have declined. Yet, it was in this period that the importance of examining the pulse, the urine, and the value of body massage was emphasized.

The famous surgical procedure of cataract removal practised during Sushruta's time reached China through Buddhist monks and pilgrims and not through Ayurvedic physicians. By the beginning of the twentieth century, it was described again but was carried out more by barber surgeons than by practitioners of Ayurveda. The practice of surgery fell into disrepute or was disregarded by Ayurveds, who preferred only to heal by medicine.

Even so, a documented performance of rhinoplasty (for which Sushruta was famous) was witnessed and recorded in Pune in 1793. A Parsee gentleman by the name of Mr Cowasjee, living in Pune, had been a bullock cart driver for the English army in the Mysore War of 1792. He was captured by the soldiers of Tipu Sultan and had his nose and one hand cut off. After one year, he and his colleague who had met the same fate sought help from a man who was known to be an expert in this field. It is believed that the person Cowasjee consulted was not an Ayurved surgeon but a bricklayer. The bricklayer gave him a new nose. Thomas Cruso and James Findlay, senior surgeons in the Bombay Presidency, witnessed the successful surgery performed by the bricklayer. They described and drew the cheek and forehead flap procedure, which was published in the *Madras Gazette*.

This surgery was subsequently reviewed in the October 1794 issue of the *Gentleman's Magazine* in London. This issue gave a full-length description of the procedure. The spectacular story caught the attention of Dr J. C. Carpue, a thirty-year-old surgeon in London. He successfully used the same flap procedure for a nose repair on one of his patients in 1814. He reported his successful results in 1816, introducing the Hindu surgical technique and with it the Indian nose to the West.

The Spread of Ayurveda

The spread of Indian learning, in particular the practice of medicine and surgery to Europe and other countries is of considerable interest. Sanskrit literature, in particular scientific texts, were translated into Pahlavi during the Sassanian reign in Persia. Khusro Nausherawan (531–579 CE) secretly sent his physician Barzoi to India. Barzoi, known as Burzuya in Pahlavi and Buzurjmihr in Persian, lived in India for many years and is believed to be none other than Vararuchi, one of the esteemed ministers of the legendary King Vikramaditya. On his return to Persia, Barzoi brought with him many Sanskrit manuscripts on medicine and other sciences, which were translated into Pahlavi. The Ayurvedic medical texts were also translated into Tibetan, Burmese, and Sinhalese, thereby spreading this system of medicine to neighbouring countries.

The early Abbasid Caliphate also promoted the translation of the *Charaka Samhita* and *Sushruta Samhita* into Arabic. In fact, a number of Indians served as royal physicians and superintendents of hospitals in Baghdad. Avicenna and Rhazes, the great Arab physicians of the Middle Ages, translated these texts into Latin, so that they now reached Europe and spread to various European countries, in particular to Italy and Spain.

Techniques in plastic surgery practised in India must have almost certainly reached Italy and Sicily by the early fifteenth century. They remained forgotten for another 450 years, until it fell to the good fortune of the English surgeon Carpue (who used Sushruta's flap procedure on his own patient) to introduce plastic surgery in Europe in the early nineteenth century.

Ayurvedic medicine suffered an eclipse after the colonization of India by the British. By 1835, state-funded medical colleges in the country taught only Western medicine and the teachings of Ayurveda were at a low ebb. Following the independence of India in 1947, Ayurveda has been re-established and rehabilitated. Even so, large urban centres increasingly practise Western medicine. There are well over one hundred Ayurvedic colleges recognized by the government—many affiliated to universities. Ayurvedic training now includes basic courses in anatomy, physiology, public health and family planning. The practice of Ayurveda in this age has incorporated a number of features of Western medicine, including the use of antibiotics, injections of various drugs and other medications found in Western pharmacopeia. This has offended many purists who feel that the ancient system of Indian traditional medicine should not be mixed with Western traditions and allopathy. I, however, cannot help but feel that its future lies in amalgamating the best of old traditions and some of the invaluable modern methodology, technology and science that characterize Western medicine.

Faith and Medicine

The importance of faith and healing has been recognized since antiquity. In ancient Greece, numerous cures and miracles were said to have been performed in Aesculapian temples— all attributed to Aesculapius, the god of healing. Cures and miracles were recorded on tablets that hung on the walls of these temples. In current times, Lourdes in France is a place of pilgrimage where sick people from all over the world seek relief from suffering and disease. Here again, faith in the Virgin Mary is reported to have led to cures often recorded as miracles. These have been accessed and carefully evaluated by eminent practitioners of Western medicine and no scientific explanation for these miraculous cures has been forthcoming.

The psyche of the average Indian, particularly in rural areas of the country, is governed by an irreplaceable faith in prayer and religion. Pilgrims visit temples, mosques, churches and dargahs in different parts of the country, particularly those known for their healing powers. They travel hundreds of miles from their towns and villages in the hope that the pilgrimage helps to preserve health or counter disease. There is also immense faith in holy men, spiritual healers and the wearing of talismans to help restore health. Faith in the healing power of prayer stretches back to antiquity. Let me quote from the scriptures (Avesta) of the ancient Persian civilization say,

> Of all the healers, Oh Spitama Zarathustra, mainly those who heal with the knife, with herbs, and with sacred incantation, the last one is the most potent as he heals from the very source of diseases.

Indeed, even today, there are many like me who believe that 'More things are wrought by prayer than this world dreams of'.

In the doctor–patient relationship, faith in the doctor unquestionably helps in healing, particularly in a critical illness. Any doctor practising any system of medicine for a significant length of time will vouch for this fact. How does faith act? Faith acts through the mind–body complex. Though there is a great deal of research going on in relation to the mind–body complex, there is very little we know and much to be learnt. The current physiological explanation is that faith acts on the mind so as to result in the stimulation of centres that control the neuroendocrine system, which release hormones and nervous impulses that help in the healing process. The centres controlling the neuroendocrine system also orchestrate the immune system of the body. A stimulation of the immune system in an integrated manner and in the right direction plays an important role in the healing process.

Indeed, faith transcends all medical systems; it reinforces the art and science of healing.

Ayurveda and Allopathy

Before I conclude, I would like to compare and contrast Ayurveda, the most important traditional system of medicine in India, with Western medicine or allopathy, perhaps now better termed as modern biomedicine.

Both Ayurveda and Western medicine have philosophical roots. The philosophical tenets expounded by Charaka in his *Charaka Samhita* have already been explained earlier. Charaka believed that these tenets would be unchanging, ever present and everlasting. Though Hippocrates is rightly considered the father of Western medicine, the philosophical roots from which Western medicine emerged came even earlier. Philosophy demanded the study of Man in all his manifold aspects, with the express purpose of devising a healthy, satisfying and happy life. Pythagoras of Samos (*ca.* 580–489 BCE), known today in particular for enunciating the Pythagoras theorem in geometry over 2,500 years ago, was the first to use the term 'philosophy' in this context. Pythagoras left Samos because of the tyranny of its ruler, Polycrates. Pythagoras founded the Italic School of Philosophy along the southern coast of Italy and lived in a small town called Croton in southern Italy, which already had a medical school. Before Pythagoras, the concept of disease was shrouded in magical and supernatural belief. After the philosophical outlook and influence of Pythagoras and the other philosophers who joined his school, disease required a rational explanation. Rational thinking and the beginnings of science were injected into the medical school.

Both Ayurveda and Hippocratic medicine believed in the 'humour theory', where a disturbance in the humours was believed to result in disease. Ayurveda continues to believe in this theory, while Western medicine has outgrown it and has negated it for several centuries.

The Hippocratic Oath detailing the duties and ethical conduct of a doctor in relation to his patients is remarkably similar to the ethical code written in the *Charaka Samhita*. Could the rules of the ethical conduct of a physician as observed in the *Charaka Samhita* have been influenced by the Greek writings of Hippocrates? Though there must have been trade and perhaps other contacts between Greece and India, notably following Alexander the Great's invasion of India, history suggests that they were independently formalized.

Ayurveda always had a holistic approach to medicine, and this, presumably, remains so. Western medicine claims to be holistic, but is clearly not so. In fact, it has become increasingly compartmentalized so that physicians treat organ systems rather than treating the patient as a whole. Modern biomedicine has not only specialists dealing with just one organ system but super specialists and super-duper specialists. As a wiseacre remarked, 'They know more and more about less and less until they know everything about next to nothing!'

In a poor, developing country such as India, medicine is influenced by economics. In fact, economics and medicine influence each other. Ayurvedic medicine is comparatively cheap, more easily affordable than Western medicine, the cost of which has often spelt financial ruin not just to poor but also to middle-class families. After all, herbs, leaves, roots and other products existing in nature constitute the mainstay of Ayurvedic medicine; by and large, these have been known and used for different ailments for centuries. Western medicine is expensive because of the research and the formulation of drugs more often designed in laboratories and manufactured by large pharmaceutical companies, and also because of the expensive technology that Western medicine necessitates.

I would like to make just one more observation related to these systems of medicine: from the nineteenth century to the first quarter of the twentieth century, Ayurveda had more drugs to offer than Western medicine. There were few cures but there were many Ayurvedic drugs that could offer relief to various problems afflicting us. What did Western medicine offer at this period of time? It could offer digitalis for dropsy, colchicine for gout, quinine for malaria, salicylates for fever and opium for pain. Treatment in Western medicine right up to the first quarter of the twentieth century chiefly consisted of causing the patient to purge, sweat and starve. Bloodletting was believed to be a panacea for almost all diseases; many a great, distinguished individual died because of this unfortunate therapy. However, after the first third of the twentieth century, and particularly in the last fifty years, Western medicine has made incredible strides. Science and technology have changed the face of medicine, so that medicine has performed miracles that would have been deemed incredible half a century back.

How did this happen? It is because the Western world was seized with the spirit of scientific inquiry. This spirit surfaced with the Renaissance (15th and 16th centuries), progressed with increasing speed and momentum up to the present, and almost certainly will continue to do so in the future. It led to discoveries in the physical sciences by great individuals such as Newton, Kepler, Galileo, Lavoisier, Mendel, Darwin, Curie, Roentgen, Einstein, Planck and a host of other great physicists, chemists, biologists and geneticists. This was soon accompanied and followed by discoveries in the medical field. To start with, there was Andreas Vesalius of the Renaissance period, whose anatomic dissections exploded the theories and mistakes of Galen that had kept medicine in chains for over a thousand years. Then came Leonardo da Vinci with his sketches of the human anatomy; Harvey, who discovered the circulation of blood; Pasteur, who proved that micro-organisms caused diseases and introduced vaccination as a prevention for disease; Koch, who discovered the tubercle bacillus; Morton, who discovered general anaesthesia; Virchow, the father of modern pathology; Lister, who introduced antisepsis and asepsis in surgery; and several others—too numerous to name. The remarkable feats in surgery of current biomedicine are known to all; they are indeed astounding and need no recounting.

And how did Ayurveda fare during this period? The artistic and cultural renaissance in India during the Gupta dynasty bypassed Ayurveda. After 1000 CE, and in particular during the latter half of the eighteenth, nineteenth and twentieth centuries, Ayurveda fell into a mire; it fell asleep. India lacked that spirit of scientific inquiry so well observed in the West. I cannot pinpoint a definite reason for this; some believe that it was the colonization of India by the British, who only encouraged Western medicine. I do not think this is wholly true. Fruitful scientific inquiry requires a conducive social, political and cultural milieu, and I believe that it was an absence of this milieu, which contributed to why India, and, for that matter, many countries in the East lag behind the West.

In spite of all that I have said, I cannot help feeling that the average Indian, the Indian in rural areas, the Indian living in slums of large cities, the poor, the marginalized, or even the middle-class Indian, deserves a better deal with regard to his health. I just cannot imagine how the deprived Indian bears his lot with such indomitable courage, fortitude and philosophical equanimity. Perhaps it is due to his religious faith, his belief and trust in God, his belief in Karma or in the immortality of his soul that enables him to do so.

The Bhagavad Gita states:

Never the spirit was born; the spirit shall cease to be never;
Never was time it was not; End and Beginning are dreams!
Birthless and deathless and changeless remaineth the spirit forever;
Death has not touched it at all, dead though the house of it seems!

This is what lies buried in the collective consciousness of the Indian mind. It is this inborn feeling that gives the average Indian strength and enables him to weather the vicissitudes of life. Must we not change this state of affairs? The poor Indian, wherever he may be, needs good sanitation, clean water, good housing, nutrition, electricity and education—particularly education for girls. He deserves to be vaccinated against diseases; needs to be better informed with regard to the preservation of health and the prevention of disease.

Traditional medicine cannot cure meningitis, severe pneumonia, a perforated viscus, fulminant sepsis, or multi-drug-resistant tuberculosis. It cannot treat HIV infection and numerous other fulminant diseases that pockmark the history of Man. Ayurveda, for example, has no answer to cancer, severe hypertension, vascular diseases, and hepatic or renal failure. The explosion of surgery and surgical techniques that characterize modern biomedicine has not even touched the traditional Indian systems of medicine.

Perhaps a day will come in the distant future when the best aspects of all systems of medicine and medical practices will be amalgamated and presented to the world as one unified system, embodying the art and science of healing—a 'Universal Medical Code'. This is a utopian, futuristic dream. We cannot however await this future. We need to act in the present, notwithstanding the difficulties in our path. Let Ayurveda and other traditional systems flourish and continue to afford relief. Yet, at the same time, it is vital, incumbent and absolutely necessary on medical, ethical and moral grounds that the fellow citizens of our country are offered at least some measure of the fruits of modern science and technology so as to help preserve better health and counter disease.

6

The Lady with the Lamp

Well past the middle of the nineteenth century, hospitals were a monumental disgrace to medicine. Hospital mortality was horrendous; death stalked the wards of hospitals in all urban centres in Europe. Hospital gangrene (the French called it *pourriture d'hôpital*) often broke out in epidemic form, as did infectious diseases like erysipelas, typhoid, cholera and dysentery. A patient was far likely to recover from illness if he or she stayed at home than if he or she ventured into a hospital, and the mortality of surgery performed on a patient at home was three or four times less than when in hospital. This sorry state of affairs exercised the minds of many thinking individuals. In the eighteenth century, John Howard had shocked the conscience of the literate with his book *Hospitals and Lazarettos*. It is remarkable that even in that era, the discerning proclaimed that infections, contagious diseases and the associated high mortality were directly related to hospitals. The surgeon Eric Erichsen believed that it was the hospital building or its atmosphere that was responsible for erysipelas and other infectious diseases. Amazingly, the concept of nosocomial infections had been grasped by some discerning individuals nearly three centuries earlier.

An important reason for the sorry state of hospitals in that era was poor nursing. And then Florence Nightingale (1820–1910) walked into history; known as 'the lady with the lamp', she lit her way into the hearts of the very many she nursed, and established the profession of nursing as we know it today. Nursing, of course, did not begin with Florence Nightingale. The urge to care for or nurse must have existed from prehistoric times. Though nursing was disorganized and rather rudimentary in the early centuries, by about the second century CE, the great Charaka had a perfect concept of the qualifications for a nurse: 'knowledge of the manner in which drugs should be prepared or compounded for administration, cleverness, devotedness to the patient waited upon, and purity (both of mind and body)'.

Nursing, today, promptly conjures a vision of gentle caring women. This is indeed true; women have always formed the core of this profession. Yet, in the Middle Ages, men tended to the sick in the hospital. During the Crusades, the Hospitallers of St John, the Teutonic Knights, and the Knights of St Lazarus, nursed the wounded and sick, as did the mendicant orders of St Francis and St Dominic.

With the rise and spread of Christianity, nursing became closely associated with various religious orders linked to the church. Perhaps the oldest religious order devoted exclusively to nursing was that of the Augustinian Nuns in the Hôtel-Dieu of Paris. The association of nursing with the church was such that even in hospitals that were totally unconnected with religion or were perhaps even irreligious, the nurses were called 'sisters'. The Reformation, an anti-Catholic movement that spread through many countries in Europe, severed the connection between nursing and the Catholic religious orders. The dedicated free service of secular religious groups was now replaced by hired workers who lacked motivation, dedication and care. Nursing in the true sense of the word was non-existent, and hospitals, as mentioned earlier, became charnel houses, breeding infections, disease and death. The Enlightenment of the eighteenth century to an extent brought back a humanitarian approach to the care of the sick. But then came the Industrial Revolution, with industry offering tempting wages to men, women and children. The clock turned back once again. Comparatively, the income from nursing was poor. To the uncaring and undedicated, nursing besides being unlucrative was demanding, repulsive and demeaning, so that the inducement to take up nursing as a wage-earning profession ceased altogether. There was indeed a dire need to improve the quality and training of nurses.

In 1840, Elizabeth Fry (1780–1845), an English Quaker, founded the Society of the Protestant Sisters of Charity, sending nurses to the homes of the sick, as also to prisons to tend to the sick. Theodor Fliedner (1800–64) and his wife Friederike were impressed by the work of Elizabeth Fry. Back in Germany, they first organized nursing care for female prison convicts and then for the sick poor. Finally, they acquired a two-hundred-bed hospital in Kaiserswerth, staffed without pay by the deaconesses of the church. The deaconesses were trained by physicians over a three-year period to become proficient in all aspects of nursing. By the time of Fliedner's death, the Kaiserswerth school had trained over fifteen hundred nurses ready to shoulder the onerous responsibility of nursing care. Elizabeth Fry had visited Kaiserswerth and had been inspired by Fliedner's work. She was the first to found the Institute of Nursing in London in 1840. Those who joined were called the 'Protestant Sisters of Charity'. There were protests that this title carried religious overtones and the name was changed to 'Sisters of Charity'. Nursing sisters, unlike those in Kaiserswerth, had received no formal instructions and were only trained in home nursing. There were others who initiated attempts to train nurses and organize the profession but none so brilliant, so gifted and so dedicated as Florence Nightingale. The history of modern nursing and the establishment of the nursing profession as we see it today is the history of the life and work of Nightingale.

* * *

Florence Nightingale was from a wealthy, cultured family. She was named Florence because she was born during the family's holiday in Florence. She was a shy but intense and stubborn girl who had set her heart as a young girl on serving mankind through nursing the sick. It is believed that on one occasion she had a visitation from God and was told that her mission in life was to serve mankind. Nursing became an obsession, a magnificent obsession. In that era, Victorian norms dictated that a woman's place was in the home, looking after the family and marrying and rearing children. Nightingale refused to be cloistered with her mother and sisters at home and insisted on following the dictates of her conscience.

Her parents, at first, forbade her to be a nurse; nursing was considered an undignified and unworthy profession for a girl from a respectable family. 'We are ducks,' cried her despairing mother, 'who have hatched a wild swan'. Nightingale stood firm. When she was twenty-one-years old, her parents relented and allowed her to visit and train at Kaiserswerth. She left Kaiserswerth after three months and went on to spend some time with the Daughters of Charity in Paris. In 1853, she returned to London and was appointed superintendent at the Establishment of Gentlewomen during Illness. She then became a superintendent of Nursing at King's College Hospital, London.

In March 1854, Britain and France declared war against Russia after the latter invaded the European provinces of the Turkish Empire, leading to the Crimean War. In September of the same year, the Allies invaded the Russian Crimean peninsula with the objective of destroying the Russian naval base at Sebastopol. They succeeded in doing so only after suffering dreadful casualties, peace being declared in 1856. Amazingly, it was the death and destruction of war that gave Florence Nightingale the occasion and opportunity to fulfil her dream to serve mankind. At the English base at Scutari hospital, conditions were dreadful. The main hospital in Scutari (now Üsküdar) was the Barrack Hospital. Of the sixty thousand British troops in the war, twenty-one thousand perished. However only 4,500 died of war wounds, the rest were dying of disease after admission to hospital.

For the first time in the history of war, there was a war correspondent from *The Times*, Thomas Chenery, reporting on events in the war zone. He reported on the pitiful conditions of the wounded and the sick in the Barrack Hospital and other hospitals in Scutari. He reported that 'Not only are there not sufficient surgeons—that, it might be urged, was unavoidable—not only are there no dressers and nurses—that might be a defect of system for which no one is to blame—but what will be said when it is known that there is not even linen to make bandages for the wounded?' The reports in the *The Times* and other newspapers led to a hue and cry in Britain. The nation was scandalized, and there was great public indignation that wounded British soldiers were attended to by untrained orderlies and dying by the hundreds because of lack of proper medical care. In contrast, the French soldiers were being cared for by the Catholic Sisters of Charity. The British Corps was accused of gross negligence. In their paper 'Nightingale in Scutari: Her Legacy Reexamined' (2005), Christopher and Gillian Gill summarize how this led to the conservative government coming under public and political pressure, prompting Sir Sidney Herbert, the Secretary of War, to make an appeal to Nightingale to lead a team of nurses to Crimea and help retrieve the desperate situation. She was chosen because her experience, dedication and managerial skills as Superintendent of Nursing at King's College, London, were well recognized. Gill & Gill mention how, remarkably on her own initiative, Nightingale had already written to her friends in Parliament volunteering her services in Crimea.

And thus it was that in November 1854, Nightingale reached Crimea with a team of thirty-eight nurses and started work at the massive Barrack Hospital in Scutari. The winter of 1854–55 was particularly horrific for the soldiers in the hospital. Florence found the conditions were even far worse than what had been reported by the war correspondents. Two thousand sick and wounded soldiers were housed in beds almost touching each other in rat-infested, poorly ventilated wards with dreadful sanitation. Dirty beds, filthy clothes, poor nutrition and food, unchanged blood-soaked bandages, no equipment for proper care, and a callous neglect towards the wounded and sick made a mockery of the word 'hospital'. The floors were filthy, leaking sewage; the walls damp and unclean; the air putrid with the smell of rotting wounds and decaying flesh. Closed windows and lack of ventilation made matters doubly worse. Lice were crawling all over the place and were aplenty in the clothes and unwashed bodies of the soldiers. This was what Florence and her team encountered when they first set foot in Barrack Hospital.

Gill & Gill illustrate the full extent of this horrific state of affairs by quoting Sarah Terrot, one of Nightingale's nurses, who recounted the following incident:

> One poor fellow neglected by the orderlies because he was dying…was very dirty, covered with wounds, and devoured by lice. I pointed this out to the orderlies, whose only excuse was, 'It's not worthwhile to clean him: he's not long for this world.' The men in bed on each side of him told me his state was such that lice swarmed from him to them.

As mentioned earlier, more soldiers died of disease than of battle wounds. Typhoid, typhus, malaria, cholera, dysentery and respiratory infections were rampant killers. The extreme crowding in the wards, the very poor sanitation and the total absence of hygiene was ideal for the spread of infections and infectious diseases. For these reasons, intestinal infections were devastating, associated with a high mortality. Gill & Gill state, 'At least three outbreaks of cholera occurred during the war: between April and September 1855, a total of 2,368 patients with cholera were admitted to one of the Scutari hospitals, of whom 1,423 (60%) died. For these patients, tincture of opium was the best treatment medical science had to offer.'

We must remember, as Gill & Gill also mention in their paper, that the Crimean war occurred twenty years before Pasteur and Koch proved that infections were caused by micro-organisms and that a particular micro-organism was responsible for a particular disease. Medicine really was primitive, for other than quinine for malaria and salicylates to temporarily reduce the degree of fever, there were no specific drugs for specific infectious diseases. There was thus an unfortunate but ready excuse given by the medical officers to explain the mortality and dreadful state of affairs in the military hospitals in Scutari.

It has been necessary to give a cogent description of the state of affairs in the hospitals in Scutari, particularly in the main Barrack Hospital, so that one realizes the formidable task facing the nursing team headed by Florence Nightingale. Speaking on the desperate situation confronting her, Nightingale said, 'The British High Command had succeeded in creating the nearest thing to hell on earth'. Amazingly, in the beginning the nurses were not even allowed to treat the dying men; they were only instructed to clean the hospital. Eventually, the number of casualties entering the hospital was so overwhelming that the nurses were allowed to help with the sick and the dying.

Florence and her nurses felt that the principal objective was to instil hygiene in every sense of the word into hospital and patient management. She is quoted as saying, 'The strongest will be wanted at the washtub'. There were no towels, basins, or soap, and only fourteen baths for two thousand soldiers. One of Nightingale's first purchases was two hundred Turkish towels. Gill & Gill provide a detailed description of the changes Nightingale implemented:

> She and her nurses washed and bathed the soldiers, laundered their linens, gave them clean beds to lie in. ...She helped establish a rational system for receiving and triaging the injured soldiers. As the wounded soldiers disembarked, they were stripped of their blood- and offal-soaked uniforms, and their wounds were bathed. To prevent cross-contamination between soldiers, Nightingale insisted that a fresh, clean cloth be used for each soldier. ...She set up huge boilers to destroy lice. ...She shamed hospital orderlies into removing buckets of human waste, to clean up the raw sewage that polluted the wards, and to unplug latrine pipes. At her behest, new windows capable of opening were installed to air out the wards. She established a separate kitchen in Barracks Hospital, which was supported by her own finances...to supplement the army's meagre rations. In response to rampant

petty corruption that was siphoning off medical supplies, she established a parallel supply system for critical materials and food, and she proved that the official supplies were being stolen by sending her representatives into the Turkish markets to buy back purloined goods. ...And significantly, she kept meticulous records of everything she saw or did.

With singular devotion and dedication, and in spite of the chauvinistic opposition to her work by senior army officers, Nightingale transformed this hellhole into a clean, properly ventilated hospital. The soldiers were now well cared for with regard to diet, cleanliness, medication and the careful dressing of wounds.

Florence Nightingale worked tirelessly, endlessly caring for the sick and wounded, and motivated the nurses in her team to do likewise. She took her last rounds of the day from bed to bed in the stillness of the night with the aid of a night lamp, ensuring that each soldier in the ward was well cared for. She was indeed the 'lady with the lamp'. The death rate in the hospital fell from 40 per cent to 2 per cent. The soldiers loved her for they promptly recognized (as most sick people do) that here was one who truly cared. One of these soldiers is known to have said, 'We lay there by hundreds; but we could kiss her shadow as it fell and lay our heads on the pillow again, content'.

It is of interest that political changes in Britain indirectly helped Florence Nightingale's work in Crimea. After the disastrous winter of 1854–55 (the first winter following the outbreak of war), there was a public outrage and parliamentary furore over the desperate state of the army and over the miserable care of wounded soldiers. The conservative coalition government led by Lord Aberdeen was forced to resign and a liberal government led by Lord Palmerston came into power. Lord Palmerston promptly sent a civil sanitary commission with instructions to improve sewers, water supply and ventilation in hospitals and camps in Scutari and in Crimea. The previous government had lacked interest in these matters and had sacked the sanitary reformer Edwin Chadwick in spite of Palmerstons's protests. The leader of the Crimean Sanitary Commission was Dr John Sutherland. The commission arrived in Scutari in March 1855 and felt that the hospitals were even filthier than the vilest slums in London. Sutherland and his colleagues hired workmen to improve ventilation, sewers and water supply. They broke four hundred windowpanes on their very first day in Scutari and let fresh air in. The repairing and unblocking of sewers was one task Florence and her nurses were not equipped to do. It contributed markedly to the improved sanitation that Nightingale introduced.

Gill & Gill note that the splendid work of Nightingale and her nurses was frowned upon by the top brass of the army. She faced marked antagonism and enmity. In fact the army released a massive report on the medical challenges in Scutari and did not even mention Florence Nightingale and her nurses. The army resented the implication that their administration and medical officers were responsible for the dreadful mortality in the hospitals. The chief medical officer reported—'they had everything—nothing was wanted'. This was in sharp contrast to Nightingale's report, which, in summary, stated that very little, almost nothing was available—everything was wanted. Who was to be believed? The public as also the civil government in London believed Nightingale. The incontrovertible fact that the hospital mortality fell sharply after her efforts at improved sanitation, the unquestioned love she received from the wounded soldiers, the reports in newspapers of her dedication and care towards the ill and wounded could not be refuted. She returned to London in 1856, hailed as a heroine.

After the war there was a public outcry that the government should institute a Royal Commission of Enquiry to report on the failing of the Army Medical Service. Nightingale championed this enquiry. In speaking of this enquiry in a chapter of the book *War and Medicine* (2008), Hugh Small mentions how the government asked Nightingale to use her influence with Queen Victoria and the public to overcome army resistance to this enquiry and describes how Nightingale was invited by the Queen to meet her and took this opportunity to press the need for the enquiry. Nightingale was the chief force behind this proposed enquiry and was powerful enough to dictate the terms of reference as also to nominate several members of this Commission. Small says that Lord Palmerston also requested her to write a confidential report to the cabinet on her work and her impression on the hospitals in Scutari.

The confidential report necessitated the collection of the mortality statistics in the army hospital during the Crimean war. Small describes how this brought Nightingale in touch with William Farr who was an expert in the field of medical statistics. Nightingale worked with Farr to analyse the mortality data. Remarkably enough, Nightingale in her youth, and against her parent's advice, insisted on studying mathematics under a tutor. This knowledge of mathematics served her in good stead, and Farr coached her in medical statistics. Their studies led them to conclude that the principle cause of death in the army hospitals was poor hygiene. When the Royal Commission of Enquiry was finally sanctioned and formed, Nightingale decided to make this the focal point in the public report. The blame for the dreadful hospital mortality did not rest with the army alone but also with the cabinet ministers of the government who had approved the hospitals without due consideration of sanitation requirements. This struck a sympathetic chord with the public, for public hygiene in civilian practice was also severely neglected. Small reported that many of the statistical findings shocked Nightingale. She discovered that in peacetime, soldiers in England died at twice the rate of civilians—even though they were young men in their prime. This was a shocking revelation of the poverty of conditions in the military services not only in war but also in peace.

* * *

Nightingale now thought of the brilliant idea of presenting the statistical information and data in charts. Statistics had been presented as graphics on rare occasions previously, but Nightingale deserves credit for using graphics prescriptively, persuading people of the need for social change. Nightingale's best known graphic has come to be known as the 'coxcomb'. It is a variation on the familiar pie graph and shows the number of deaths each month and the causes. Each month was represented as a twelfth of a circle. Months with more deaths were shown as larger wedges, so that the area of each wedge represented the number of deaths in that particular month. Causes of death in each of the wedges were classified into three categories—from disease, coloured blue; from wounds, coloured red; and from other causes, coloured black. The graphics (coxcomb) between April 1854 and March 1855 showed a horrendous mortality in every month, most of the mortality being due to disease. The graphics from April 1855 to March 1856 showed a sharp fall in mortality; even so, the major portion of the mortality still was due to disease and not from wounds. Nightingale preferred the coxcomb graphic to the conventionally used bar graph because it allowed a more easy comparison in mortality in each month of the year—between 1854–55 and 1855–56. Also the coloured coxcomb graphic was more arresting to the eye. Nightingale said her coxcomb graphic was designed to 'affect thro' the eyes what we may fail to convey to the brains of the public through their word-proof ears'.

When the report of the Royal Commission was published in 1858, it had an appendix that contained the graphical representation of statistics detailing rather picturesquely (through the coxcomb) the causes of the observed mortality in British Crimean hospitals. Disease, rather than war wounds, was the major killer and the cause stated by the Commission was poor hygiene. This had a great impact on the lay public. There also was a transfer of experience from the Crimean war to preventive medicine in civilian practices. This came about solely because of the government's decision to send Nightingale to Crimea and then ask her to orchestrate a public enquiry into the treatment of the sick and wounded in the army-managed hospitals in Scutari. She became a heroine, an iconic figure who could lend her name and fame to the sanitarian movement that had been stalled by the removal of Edwin Chadwick, a sanitarian who for years had championed the importance of hygiene in public health.

Nightingale brought the sanitary lessons of the Crimean War to the civil population through village committees, home nursing visits and other initiatives, resulting in a remarkable improvement in hygienic standards. She wrote and distributed pamphlets on the role and importance of hygiene, as also popular books, the most important of which was *Notes on Nursing: What It Is and What It Is Not* (1859), a self-help manual for laypeople. Her crusade for improved civilian sanitation occupied much more of her time over the next fifteen years after the war than her previous interest in hospital nursing.

Nightingale was also engaged in major projects. She was largely responsible in setting up the first major military medical school in London. She played an important role in hospital design and construction in the post–Crimean War period; her book *Notes on Hospitals* (1859) was the standard text on this subject. She was the guiding spirit in the reconstruction of St Thomas Hospital and many other hospitals in Britain and in other countries. Her architectural views on the medical aspects governing the construction of hospitals were put into effect during these projects. A public appeal to start a nursing school under Florence Nightingale brought in £44,000, and her first batch of students graduated from her school at St Thomas in 1861. Her objective was to train matrons—these graduates would then in turn train new recruits into nurses who could join hospitals. She managed thereby to prise the management of nursing and nurses from the supervision of hospital deans, placing them under the control of matrons. Her nursing matrons spread far and wide both in the West and the East spreading her gospel to several countries of the world. Her book *Notes on Nursing* became compulsory reading for all those who joined the nursing profession. The stress in her teachings was always on basic hygiene, and in the book she says, 'Nursing has been limited to signify little more than the administration of medicines and the application of poultices. It ought to signify the proper use of fresh air, light, warmth, cleanliness, quiet, and the proper selection and administration of diet'.

The stress of Nightingale's work in Crimea, her organizing, travelling, writing and working long hours inevitably took a toll on her health. She suffered a number of illnesses, perhaps a series of nervous breakdowns. Her health was particularly fragile after she suffered a serious febrile illness (perhaps typhoid) in Crimea, but she continued to write extensively and work tirelessly.

* * *

Several contemporary historians have levelled criticisms against Nightingale, mentioning that she was a little more than a manager with little talent for patient care. These characterizations are untrue, unkind and a total travesty of accepted historical facts. A recent (2009) article in *Historia Medicinae* by Rosemary Leadbeater titled 'Florence Nightingale: Nursing, Lifestyle, and Her Influence on and Inter-relationships with Women' finds fault with Nightingale's approach to the identity of women and her philosophy on obedience within the wider context of her management of nurse training, her life and apparent breakdown, and her relationships with her associates.

Leadbeater concedes that Nightingale was a feminist; her many writings support her feminist fervour. However, she purports that in Nightingale's view women should deploy their skills as nurses rather than as doctors. Leadbeater claims Nightingale did not encourage women to break into the medical profession. Had she done so, many more women would have stepped out of the narrow confines of their Victorian upbringing. In fact, she actively condemned women such as Elizabeth Blackwell, the first qualified woman doctor in the United States, who with Elizabeth Garrett in Britain was campaigning for women to break into medicine. Leadbeater claims that Nightingale was also not particularly supportive of the women's rights activists of the day and was indifferent to women's suffrage. She was therefore a feminist only when it came to nursing, unsupportive of and even opposing the advance of women in other fields of human endeavour.

A further criticism levelled by this author is that Nightingale insisted on the nurse being completely obedient to the doctor, linking the necessary compliance of the nurse to that of the soldier. She could not break away from the rigidness of some Victorian beliefs. Leadbeater also suggests that Nightingale's priorities lay with the 'micro-management of nurses' lives rather than on professional training, focusing on their lifestyle and their moral conduct rather than their development of technical skills'. Her illness and frequent nervous breakdowns have also excited criticism from Leadbeater. She claims that Nightingale's illness was a ruse to allow her to work undisturbed, receiving only the visitors she chose, and that it was an efficient way to maximize her time and energy. Lytton Strachey in his work *Eminent Victorians* (1918) also writes on the effectiveness of

Nightingale's illness and says, 'She found the machinery of illness hardly less effective as a barrier against the eyes of men than the ceremonial of a palace'. Leadbeater goes even one step further and comments that evidence suggests that Nightingale's illness was spurious, and as long as it continued, it provided her with the means to control her associates.

Many of these comments are decidedly unfair and need to be rebutted. Nightingale was a Victorian, born and bred in an upper-class Victorian environment. The remarkable fact is that she broke the shackles of her environment, stepped out of the confines of her upper-class female submissive role to blaze a new trail—the founding of modern nursing. It is quite likely that her Victorian upbringing demanded strict discipline and obedience from her nurses and that she valued the importance of good character in those who entered the nursing profession. This probably prompted her to monitor the lifestyles of her trainee nurses. Though emancipated from many strict Victorian traditions, she may not have been sufficiently emancipated to champion women's suffrage or fight for women's rights.

It is obvious that Nightingale's life's mission was to serve humanity—to start with, it was to nurse the sick, which she so effectively and efficiently did in Scutari, and then to establish nursing as a profession not only in her own country but in many countries of the world, far and wide. As mentioned earlier, she championed along with others the importance of good sanitation and was indirectly responsible for saving many civilian lives, thereby increasing the life expectancy in Britain during the tenure of her work. All her time and energies were focused towards these difficult tasks. It would perhaps have been impossible to take on other onerous responsibilities in relation to the further enfranchisement of women, even if she had the desire and inclination to do so.

Unquestionably, Nightingale was in frail health. Imagine the arduousness of her work in Crimea under difficult, dreadful conditions followed by her continuous activities on her return to her country. A state of nervous exhaustion is perpetuated if one continues to expend energy without resting. It is possible that she used her frail health to allow her to work undisturbed and in seclusion, rather than to expose herself to the rigours of an active public life. It is more than likely that her design of hospitals, the training of matrons in nursing school, and her numerous writings were only possible because she secluded herself and restricted those wanting to meet her. Leadbeater picks on what she considers to be Nightingale's failings, not realizing that her virtues and her accomplishments far outweigh these failings. Her criticisms lack a sense of an overall perspective.

Not many realize that Nightingale's work has had far-reaching effects. Gill & Gill claim that she has influenced at least three areas of contemporary medicine—I have summarized their claims in the following paragraphs.

The first area Nightingale contributed to was the concept of hospital infection control. The authors say:

Many of our current health care practices, such as isolation of patients with antibiotic-resistant pathogens, avoidance of cross contamination, routine cleansing of all patient areas, aseptic preparation of foods, ventilation of wards, and disposal of human and medical wastes, trace their origins to practices enacted by Nightingale at Scutari.

Remarkably enough, the backdrop of the Crimean War indirectly served to help the sanitarian movement against the prevailing medical dogma, which paid little attention to hygiene and to the importance of prevention of disease. Nightingale did not originate sanitarian ideas and theories. It was Chadwick who did so, but the impact of her well published work and reforms in the hospitals in Crimea gave a great boost to the sanitation movement. It also changed the treatment of hospitalized and infected patients in civilian hospitals. To quote Nightingale's words, 'In the present (so-called) enlightened time, sound principles of Hygiene are by no means widely spread even among the civil medical profession. To this circumstance it appears mainly to be owing that the belief in contagion as an unavoidable cause of death from epidemic disease is still so prevalent'.

Though civilian health improved from the lessons learnt in the Crimean War, it is difficult to quantify this improvement. It has been clearly shown that the life expectancy in Britain increased from thirty-nine years at the end of the war to fifty-five years at the time of Nightingale's death in 1920, this being one of the steepest rises in medical history. There is evidence that this rise was not related to vaccination, medical treatment, or decrease in the virulence of microbes. There is a strong belief that the two main reasons for this remarkable increase in life expectancy were improved sanitation and hygiene together with improved nutrition. Nightingale was an important public figure who resuscitated this sanitarian movement through her work in Scutari. Her public stature following her return from Crimea helped to entrench this movement as an important feature of government policy.

The second field influenced by Nightingale is hospital epidemiology. Her early training in mathematics was further influenced by the work of Adolphe Quetelet (1796–1874), the leading statistician of the day. The authors quote the following annotations that Nightingale made in her copy of Quetelet's book: 'All Sciences of Observation depend upon Statistical methods—without these, are blind empiricism. Make your facts comparable before deducing causes. Incomplete, pell-mell observations arranged so as to support theory, insufficient number of observations, this is what one sees'. The elegance of her statistical diagrams illustrating the causes of deaths in the Crimean War were not just descriptive—they were, more importantly, prescriptive, pointing out the methods that needed to be prescribed to reduce this mortality.

Finally, there are some historians who argue that hospice medicine is indebted to Nightingale. As a nurse looking after seriously ill soldiers, Nightingale helped many to survive and yet by her own account closed the eyes of hundreds. One of the duties she assigned to herself was to write letters to the families of patients who were dead or dying, explaining the circumstances of their death and often enclosing some of these soldiers' personal effects to their families.

Therefore, notwithstanding some of the criticisms levelled against her, there is little doubt that Nightingale's virtues far outweigh a few failings that she may have had in her long life. And is there a man or woman, however great he or she may be, who is without a few failings? Nightingale indeed was a great woman. She owed her success to her obsessive motivation, a vision to which she steadfastly adhered, to professional ability and competence, and to a profound devotion to her cause. She transformed nursing from lowly beginnings to a noble and highly respected profession that embodies within itself the very essence of the art of healing. She ensured that the nurse and doctor were equal partners in the fight against disease. She exemplified the care of the sick in her personal odyssey through life, and amazingly also successfully institutionalized care in the nursing profession for posterity. We quote her basic tenets that are equally applicable to the art and science of medicine—tenets that are compellingly as relevant today as they were in her day:

> The art is that of *nursing the sick*. Please mark—*nursing the sick; not* nursing sickness.... This is the reason why nursing proper can only be taught at the patient's bedside and in the sick-room or wards. Neither can it be taught by lectures or by books, though these are valuable accessories.

The lady with the lamp had cast an eternal glow on an uncaring world.

7

Music, the Mind and Medicine

There is nothing in the world so much like prayer as music is.

—WILLIAM P. MERRILL

Music is an innate feature of the human psyche. It is deeply rooted in human nature and remains a fundamental attribute and activity of the human species. Millions of people listen to music today—more than ever before in the history of the world. There is music on television, computers and the radio; music in churches and temples; music on the streets and subways; music in concert halls, theatres and opera houses; and recordings of every kind of music and musical event on compact discs, making it available to a wider range of the population than could ever have been imagined sixty or seventy years ago. Music, remarkably enough, is very often a feature of one's working day and certainly an important aspect in the lifespan of most individuals. We listen to music and we beat time to what we hear; we play music; we sing, hum, whistle; we dance and clap when music moves us to do so. Verily, the world is filled with the sound of music.

From the beginning of time, there is no culture which lacks music. Music dates from antiquity as proven by Palaeolithic cave paintings. These paintings show dancing figures. Flutes made of bone that have been found in these caves suggest that they danced to some form of music. Drawings and paintings, particularly of animals, found on the cave walls at numerous sites in Europe and other parts of the world are given prime importance as integral features of the lives and activities of Palaeolithic humans. Music, however, is so interwoven with human activity that it must have surely played a greater part in prehistory than can ever be ascertained.

What must have prompted prehistoric man to indulge in the art forms of drawing and painting? I would have thought that these primitive art forms were just an expression of their innate human nature, but most art historians differ from this view. In his book *Music and the Mind* (1992), Anthony Storr postulates that these artists painted and drew animals in order to exercise magical charms on them. Storr hypothesizes that by capturing the image of the animal on the wall of a cave, they felt they could probably control it. Drawing and painting animals enabled the Palaeolithic man to know his prey more accurately and thereby be more successful in his hunt.

Storr quotes the historian Herbert Read who wrote:

> Far from being an expenditure of surplus energy, as earlier theories have supposed, art, at the dawn of human culture, was a key to survival, a sharpening of the faculties essential to the struggle for existence. Art, in my opinion, has remained a key to survival.

The art form of literature came later in the history of mankind. It was almost certainly derived from the wandering storyteller, who not only told stories to entertain, but also recounted traditions, myths, values and moral norms that gave a coherence to society, giving each individual a sense of identity and purpose that helped him or her face the problems of life and living.

If this is indeed true, Storr poses a question that I, too, have often asked: of what use is music? Music, Storr says, is 'a form of communication between people'. But what does it communicate? It does not alter our perception of the external world nor does it convey information or knowledge as language does. Is music of practical use? Is it, as Storr suggests, a human activity that to start with was 'adaptively useful'? I do not think so. The human brain is structured to distinguish noise from music. It responds to tones, tunes, rhythm, and to different musical forms. How does this come about? Does music serve a purpose? I feel all art is an inevitable expression of an innate feature of the human psyche, an expression of an evolved attribute perhaps imprinted in the DNA of the human species. I disagree with Read that 'art was and has remained the key to survival'.

Of all the art forms in our world, in my opinion, music is the greatest. I speak of great music—music which penetrates into the very depth of a human being, transcendental music, music which enables one to commune with God.

This essay now proceeds with some thoughts on the origin, evolution and the mystery of music, followed by the effects of music on the mind, its inherent power and its relation to medicine. It concludes with a brief description on its nature and significance. I write chiefly with reference to Western music. Though familiar with all forms of Western music, my special interest is Western classical music. I am also familiar, but to a lesser extent, with Indian classical music. But the remarks that follow apply in general to all music. Different cultures and different countries have different music, and each culture by and large is most fond of music that originated and evolved within its history. But the world, figuratively speaking, is getting smaller; science and technology have increased interconnectivity between humans, communities and countries. Culturally, we get to learn and understand aspects of different civilizations. One aspect being increasingly appreciated is music of different countries. To give an example, there is increasing appreciation of Indian music in the West, just as there is increasing appreciation of Western music in India and the Far East.

Music has evolved over millennia to become complex and sophisticated. Both Western and Indian music have different art forms, ranging from the early classical to the various other modes that appeal to individuals who are not fond of the classical versions. Be that as it may, how did music begin, how did it come into the world, what is the origin of music? A knowledge of its origin would perhaps give us an idea of its fundamental meaning.

In the East, all things good, great and beautiful have the mark of divinity—they are the gifts of the gods to those on earth; and music is one such great God-given gift. Music—what we call *sangita* in Hindi, or *mausiki* in Urdu—is closely linked to philosophy and religion, and in India, philosophy and religion can explain the inexplicable. Sound is believed to be of two kinds, the vibration of ether and the vibration of air. The former is 'unstruck sound'; it corresponds to Pythagoras's 'music of the spheres'. It is inaudible to humans but has forever been the delight of the gods. The latter, the 'struck sound', corresponds to manmade music in the world. It is believed, however, 'to reflect the laws of the universe and results from the union of the physical breath with the fire of the intellect'. Tradition has it that God Brahma taught song to the legendary sage Narada, who then taught and transmitted it to mankind.

The earliest texts in Indian music are hymns and incantations grouped in the four Vedas. The Vedas are believed to have been dictated to the rishis of the ancient past by the gods.

Sung recitation was given the name of 'Vedic psalmody'. It was codified in the *Samaveda* and was a basic element in the worship that Aryans established in India after their arrival into the country around 1500 BCE.

Could there be a relation between the 'unstruck sound' (the music of the spheres, the sound of silence) of the gods and the 'struck sound' of man? I believe there may well be. Sound does not exist on its own or by itself; it has a permanent, unavoidable relation to silence. The first played or sung note of a musical composition is not the beginning; it emerges, emanates from the silence that precedes it. Equally, the last played or sung note of a musical composition is transformed back into silence. Thus the 'struck sound' or the music of man emanates from the 'unstruck sound', the music of the gods (the sound of silence), and returns from where it arose.

Metaphysically and metaphorically speaking, this is indeed a profound philosophical thought if this analogy of music is extended to life on earth. Perhaps life on earth emanates from the supreme being or power that controls and orders the universe and, in course of time, returns from where it emerged.

The Western mind does not eschew religion and philosophy but has tried to explain the origin of music through reason, inquiry and study. It has failed to do so, and even today, the origin of music is shrouded in mystery. There are many views in the West on this subject; but the fact that there are many views proves the point that there is no general agreement. Could the origin of music be linked tenuously to the sounds of nature—the sounds of running water, waterfalls, rivers? Sounds in nature, however pleasant, are irregular noises rather than the sustained tones that form music. There is a view that the origin of music may well be related to birdsong. Current research on birdsong, however, shows that birdsong does show variations in pitch, change of key and variations of a theme. The wood thrush, for example, has been shown to have a repertoire of as many as nine songs, which can be sung consecutively and in different combinations. The view that the origin of music lies in the imitation of birdsong is highly unlikely and, in my opinion, can be dismissed. For one, if human music indeed began this way, we should find examples of music resembling birdsong in primitive and pre-literate communities. Music in these communities takes the form of complex rhythmic patterns bearing no resemblance to birdsong. Also, birdsong is musically speaking very complicated and difficult to reproduce. Modern Western classical music (particularly a few works by Liszt and Dvořák) do manage to reproduce to an extent the twittering of birds. But these are highly sophisticated developments in the history of music.

Igor Stravinsky, a great modern composer of Western music, maintains that natural sounds like the murmur of the rustling of leaves in a breeze, the rippling of a brook, or birdsong may suggest music but are not in themselves so. He writes, 'I conclude that tonal elements become music only by virtue of their being organized, and that such organization presupposes 'a conscious human act'.

Music is composed of tones, which are separate units with constant auditory waveforms. Since many years, we have the technology to define the difference between tones in terms of pitch, timbre and characteristics of the waveforms. But science cannot *exactly* identify the relation between tones that constitutes music.

Could the origin of music be linked to speech? Storr offers useful information on this theory as well, which I have summarized here. Linguistic scholars distinguish the prosodic features of speech from its syntactic features. The prosodic features of speech convey pitch, volume, timbre, emphasis and emotional content, while syntactic speech is concerned with grammatical structure, syntax and literal meaning. Prosodic communication and music have significant similarities. In fact, a popular belief in the late nineteenth century was that the evolution of music consisted in the gradual separation of the prosodic elements of adult speech from its syntactic. When speech became emotional, the 'sounds' assumed a greater tonal range, as also varying pitch and timbre, thereby coming closer to 'music'. These sounds became gradually uncoupled from the words that accompanied them and came to exist as separate entities constituting the language of music.

Darwin took an opposite view and supposed that music preceded speech, arising from 'an elaboration of mating calls'. A sound used to attract the attention of a potential mate, became modified and elaborated in various ways giving rise to the basic features of tone, timbre and pitch that constitute music.

Jean-Jacques Rousseau, the father of the French revolution, and also an accomplished author and musician, believed that song preceded speech at the beginning of history. In any case, if song and speech were initially linked and with time became increasingly distinct, the differences in their functions grew to be even more accentuated. Speech was for conveying information and discussing ideas; song was for the musical communication of emotions and feelings toward individuals, as also to large audiences.

It will be impossible to establish these origins of human music with certainty. The current prevalent Western view, as reflected in the words of Storr, is that music 'originated and developed from the prosodic exchanges between mother and infant which help to foster the bond between them'. The sounds of different pitch, tone and amplitude made by the mother (denoting unconditional love) coupled with the babbling and lalling of the infant, either spontaneous or in response to the mother, may perhaps be responsible for the development of music. Storr claims that from this start, music 'became a form of communication between adult human beings. As the capacity for speech and conceptual thought developed, music became less important as a way of conveying information, but retained its significance as a way of communicating feelings and cementing bonds between individuals, especially in group situations'.

It must be remembered that for most of its history, music has been predominantly a group activity, serving an essential role in social interaction, as also serving religious and ceremonial purposes. Anthropologists have suggested that vocal music may well have been one distinctive way of communicating with the supernatural. In his Charles Eliot Norton lectures delivered at Harvard from 1939 to 1940, Stravinsky affirms, 'The profound meaning of music and its essential aim is to promote a communion, a union of man with his fellowmen and with the Supreme Being'.

Though the origins of music may be clouded in mystery, it has evolved from its earliest beginnings to a sophisticated complexity, which characterizes music of this day and age. We see, today, the compositions of great composers played by large orchestras to huge audiences in specially built concert halls. We also see individuals playing music for the sheer love of music, and individuals who may listen alone to the music they like. We are witness to the evolution of numerous different instruments that make music and the coming of age of virtuosos who perform in public on instruments that they have mastered. There is, however, no greater or more sublime instrument in the world than the human voice. A sweet, melodious, far-ranging voice is the personification of quintessential beauty in music.

I would like to briefly comment on two forms of Western music—the world of grand opera and the world of jazz. I do so because each, in its own way, is strongly emotive, powerfully affecting the psyche, the mind and—through the mind—the mind–body complex. The opera depicts on a grand stage a musical drama that is sung by different singers—some singing individually and some in combination.

What makes opera 'grand'? Why are so many addicted to it? Opera strongly dramatizes various basic aspects of life. It lays bare a slice of life, a vastly magnified cross-section of life, in our world. Opera dramatizes passions emotions; love, hate, envy, jealousy, virtue, vice, greed, charity, bravery, treachery, sacrifice, joy, tragedy are all enfolded within a dramatic story. These passions and emotions are not only pin-pointed but vastly magnified—much larger than life. Each such dramatized, magnified emotion or passion, as it enfolds in the story, is *hurled* at the audience and has an immediate impact. How is opera different from theatre? In theatre, words are spoken; in opera, words are sung by beautiful voices, loud and clear, and it is the music uncensored by the brain that directly touches and moves the heart. Opera is in many ways bigger than theatre, bigger than life, and it is music that makes it so.

The stage is, in general,
a painting of the human passions,
the original of which
is in every human heart.
—Jean-Jacques Rousseau

The world of jazz consists of a multitude of sounds ranging from the early blues to Dixieland, to swing bands, Charleston bands, and many more. Jazz is completely a player's art; it is improvisation on a theme rather than composition. This means that the player of jazz is also a composer, which points to the creativity of this music. Great jazz played by great virtuosos is indeed great music, and there are many who prefer this form of music to Western classical music. In fact jazz can be compared to great Indian music. The latter is based on ragas. Each raga consists of a seven-note mathematical scale, and the music, be it vocal or instrumental, confines itself to these seven notes, which can and have to be played in various combinations and permutations. It is indeed a remarkable form of spontaneous improvisation, so that the rendering of a particular raga by different musicians is almost never the same. There are several such ragas for several different occasions, for different seasons, and for different times of the day or night. Let me return to Western classical music. Great orchestras of the world may make beautiful music, which listeners love; yet, the greatest honour and reverence is reserved for the musicians of the past and present who have composed this music. To quote Claude Levi-Strauss: 'Since [music] is the only language with the contradictory attributes of being at once intelligible and untranslatable, the musical creator is a being comparable to the gods, and music itself the supreme mystery of the science of man'.

Music and the Mind

How does one recognize and appreciate music? This involves a bit of neurology which may be familiar to the physician but not to a layperson. Music reaches the ear in the form of sound waves. These are then channelled through the ear canal to the eardrum, causing it to vibrate. The vibrations are relayed through a chain of three small bones in the middle ear. The last of these bones is the stapes, which connects to the cochlea. The cochlea is a part of the inner ear, which is connected with hearing. It is filled with fluid, which surrounds some ten thousand to fifteen thousand hair cells termed 'cilia'. Vibrations of the stapes cause the sound waves to send fluid waves within the cochlea, leading to a vibratory movement of the cilia. These cilia are now stimulated to release neurotransmitters that activate the auditory nerve, which carries nervous impulses in the form of electrical currents to the auditory cortex in the temporal lobe of the brain.

The above explanation holds for sound waves caused by speech, any form of noise, as also musical sound waves related to music. The further appreciation of musical sound waves was till very recently a mystery. How were sound waves produced by music appreciated as music? The discovery of new imaging procedures on the brain has helped to clarify some of these issues. Studies using MRI and positron emission tomography (PET) scans suggest that there are a number of networks, perhaps interconnected with one another, that are responsible for decoding and interpreting various aspects of music. Imaging suggests that a small area of the temporal lobe recognizes pitch, which forms the basis of melody (patterns of pitch over time), chords (several pitches which sound at the same time) and harmony (two or more melodies at the same time). Another adjacent part of the brain recognizes and decodes timbre. Timbre is the quality of sound, and this part of the brain can distinguish between two or three individuals singing the same note from the difference in the timbre or quality of the sung note, just as we can distinguish between different instruments playing the same note. Current research leads us to believe that the cerebellum processes rhythm, and the emotional content of music is interpreted by the frontal lobe. Music, which is strongly emotive, is believed to light up the 'reward centre', which is a region of the hypothalamus. The same centre lights up through pleasurable stimuli produced for example, by eating chocolates or drinking alcohol.

Every human brain is wired to perform the complex task of appreciating music. There, however, has to be a difference between the average human brain with regard to the appreciation of music and that of musicians, particularly great musicians, composers, virtuosos and conductors of orchestral music. Their brains must be specially wired for their great musical memories, musical appreciation and interpretations. The virtuosos on the violin, piano, or any instrument can play several concertos from memory on the instrument each has mastered. How do they do so? There is no time for a great virtuoso, who often gives three performances or more in a week in different cities of the world, to practise the programme he is to play when the programme is different for each centre. What is he to do? Incredible as it may sound, he practises the score of the music he is supposed to play within his mind; he plays it in his mind often while commuting from one city to the other. And when the musician rehearses a concerto or a sonata in his mind, he can picture, with his mind's eye, the movement of his fingers and, if he is a violinist or cellist, also of the bow. The musical memory of great conductors, the maestros who conduct large orchestras, is even more incredible. They conduct whole symphonies, operas and concertos from memory. The whole score of each instrument in an orchestra of over a hundred musicians is within a maestro's mind; he gives the right cues to the instrument that has to come into the music, he knows every nuance, every change in rhythm and time, every accelerando and diminuendo, every pianissimo and fortissimo, the music demands. He interprets and conveys the interpretation of great music with his baton, hands, eyes, and the measured movements of his head and body. I, who am reasonably musical and play—rather indifferently—a musical instrument, find this feat nothing short of miraculous. There must be a reason for this prodigious musical memory, and we must wait for science to unravel it.

At the other end of this spectrum, there are many instances where trauma or disease afflicting the brain can cause defects in musicality. It is important to take note of these if one is to better understand the relationship between music, the mind and the brain. These defects must obviously be related to changed (disrupted or new) connections within the brain about which we are more or less ignorant. The hearing of music in rare instances can give rise to motor or sensory disorders. I shall just give a few examples of what I have stated above; for a more complete discussion, I would refer the reader to Oliver

Sacks' *Musicophilia: Tales of Music and the Brain* (2007) and to Macdonald Critchley and R. A. Henson's *Music and the Brain: Studies in the Neurology of Music* (1977), two works from which the following information has been derived.

MUSICOGENIC EPILEPSY

Musicogenic epilepsy is a rare disorder in which music triggers a seizure. It was first described in 1937 by MacDonald Critchley. The type of music that induced seizures in the eleven patients he described varied. The seizure could be of the nature of temporal lobe epilepsy or could take the form of petit mal or grand mal epilepsy. The most striking case that Critchley described was of the eminent music critic Nikonov, who had his first seizure at a performance of Meyerbeer's opera *The Prophet*. Soon any music, however soft the volume, would induce a fit. He had to give up his profession and avoid all contact with music. He developed a phobia of all music, which he described in a small pamphlet entitled 'Fear of Music'.

MUSICOPHILIA

Oliver Sacks reports a remarkably unusual case history of a man who was struck by lightning while talking to his mother on a payphone. He had a cardiac arrest and an out-of-body experience due to the arrest but was successfully resuscitated. There was a slight impairment of memory lasting for a few weeks, but he, then, felt perfectly well and on a careful neurological examination was found to be perfectly normal. He was a surgeon by profession and soon resumed work.

Six to eight weeks after his recovery from the cardiac arrest, he felt an intense desire to listen to piano music. He bought recordings of piano music and was particularly enamoured by Vladimir Ashkenazy's recordings of Chopin's works. Soon after this desire to hear piano music, he started to hear music in his head. He wanted to write down what he heard but hardly knew how to notate music. He wrestled with learning to play Chopin on the piano and also to give form to the music he continuously heard. He was convinced that the music playing in his head was not a hallucination. He termed it an 'inspiration'. Amazingly, he succeeded in playing the piano well, gave a concert where he played one of Chopin's Scherzos and played a composition of his own termed 'Rhapsody, Opus I' brilliantly—an astounding feat for someone with virtually no musical background. Oliver Sacks had no convincing explanation for this sudden musicality in his patient. Perhaps during his cardiac arrest, where he had an out-of-body experience, neural connections might have been so altered or rearranged that the eventual result was an exceptional urge for musicality.

Defects in music appreciation are not uncommon. The patient may for example not be able to discern rhythm. Sacks remarks on how Ché Guevera, the great Cuban revolutionary and the companion-in-arms of Fidel Castro, would continue to dance the steps of the mambo when the orchestra played the tango! There are some who are tone-deaf, and some who fail to recognize pitch, just as there are a few who are absolutely pitch perfect. Total amusia—the inability to recognize or reproduce musical tones—is rare; recognition of music as music is absent and the amusic individual hears music as a screeching sound.

THE MOZART EFFECT

Inspired by the observation that many musicians have excellent mathematical ability, an article in *Harvard Men's Health Watch* stated how researchers at the University of California, Irvine, studied the effect of listening to music on cognitive function and ability in general, and spatial temporal reasoning in particular. They showed with consistency that those listening for ten minutes to a Mozart sonata had better IQ scores than those who listened to relaxation tapes, or those who waited in silence. While it is not clear how exactly music enhances cognitive performance, the paper states that the researchers believe that music helps to fire neurons in the right half of the cerebral hemisphere, which is responsible for higher functions. Mozart's music helps exercise selected brain cells allowing them to process information more efficiently. The study did, however, conclude that the 'Mozart effect' is modest and temporary. Yet, the fact that perhaps some form of music can boost cognitive function is indeed of great interest and warrants further research. For example, could listening to Mozart for longer periods of time or listening to his music every day produce a more lasting improvement of cognitive function? Would suitable music of other composers, for example Chopin, Bach, or Mendelssohn, produce the same effect? If not, what is it in Mozart's music that causes this effect. Perhaps it is the simplicity and quintessential beauty to which the brain responds.

Interestingly, through another study, it has been suggested that listening to Hindustani classical instrumental music played on the santoor improved writing skills of students with learning disabilities. The authors of this study conclude that learning disabilities are neurologically based processing problems, and music stimulates the brain centres that deal with reading, writing, thinking, analysing and planning skills.

We now need to ask an important question. In which cerebral hemisphere is music decoded and appreciated? It is generally agreed that in the right-handed individual, language, leading to speech, is processed in the left cerebral hemisphere, while music is scanned and decoded in the right cerebral hemisphere. Many eminent neurologists, however, claim that it is wrong to specify an exact anatomical location within the brain for a specific neurological function and that considerable overlap exists between many cerebral functions. It is, however, the left hemisphere that deals with conceptual thought that leads to language and speech; the right hemisphere is linked with emotions as in poetry and song.

Anthony Storr has given examples that demonstrate the difference between the right and left hemispheres in a variety of ways. If for example, the left cerebral hemisphere is sedated by the injection of a barbiturate in the left carotid artery, the subject cannot speak but can yet sing. Interestingly, Storr notes that 'stammerers can sometimes sing sentences which they cannot speak; presumably because the stammering pattern is encoded in the left hemisphere, whilst the singing is predominantly a right hemispheric activity'. Above all, patients who have a disease or have suffered trauma to the left cerebral hemisphere may lose the ability to understand the symbolic significance of speech, nor make use of language, without losing the ability to comprehend and appreciate music, denoting a preservation of musical competence. Storr cites the example of a famous neuropsychologist, A. R. Luria, who studied a composer named Vissarion Shebalin. The composer suffered a stroke leading to sensory aphasia. Yet, he continued to teach music and composed his fifth symphony, which—according to musician Dmitri Shostakovich—was brilliant. Battle wounds that drastically damage the left cerebral hemisphere can affect speech, spatial perception and memory. Yet, these patients may be able to appreciate music as well as they did before the inflicted wound and can remember melody but not the words.

Finally let me quote the example of the musician portrayed in Oliver Sacks' book *The Man who mistook his Wife for a Hat: And Other Clinical Tales* (1985). This man suffered from a brain disease that, though enabling him to see, made it impossible for him to recognize the essential identity of objects, so—as the title indicates—he mistook his wife for a hat! Yet, amazingly, his musical memories were unimpaired. In fact, he could dress himself, eat a meal, or have a bath only if he was singing. His external world was in shambles, and he could only give some meaning or structure to it through music.

The Power of Music

Music has been shown to impact the intellectual, perceptual, language and literary skills, as also the personal and social development of children and young adults. This has been well-illustrated in 'The Power of Music: Its Impact on the Intellectual, Social and Personal Development of Children and Young People', a 2010 paper authored by Susan Hallam, Institute of Education, University of London.

The beneficial impact of music on the intellectual, perceptual, literary, social, and personal development of children and young adults has been an observation for several decades. Current scientific research further bears this out.

Let me start by stating that our knowledge of the working of the brain, particularly with reference to its higher functions is still in its infancy. Indeed, there is very little we know and much more we need to know. The main functional cell unit within the brain is termed the neuron. The human brain contains approximately one hundred billion neurons, many of which are active simultaneously. Recent advances in the study of the brain have helped us to understand why listening to music or 'making' music for example, by playing an instrument influences other cerebral activities. The cerebral cortex 'self-organizes' itself as one engages in either listening to music or making music. What does this mean? Susan Hallam explains that musical experiences are processed within the brain through interaction between neurons, each neuron having possibly a thousand connections with other neurons. When musical experiences are repeated frequently, the efficacy of these neuronal interconnections are both enhanced and fine-tuned over varying time scales. Intensive and active engagement with music can thus induce cortical reorganization producing functional changes on how the brain processes information. These alterations may become hardwired over time producing permanent changes in information processing.

Research suggests that the skills developed from self-organization of the cortex due to musical activities may then be transferred to other activities, if the processes involved are similar. For example, music and speech share a number of common processing systems. The enhanced processing systems within the cortex resulting from the musical experiences can therefore impact the perception of language, which—in turn—would impact the ability to learn to read.

Music and Medicine

> *The poets did well to conjoin music and medicine in Apollo, because the office of medicine is but to tune this curious harp of man's body, and to reduce it to harmony.*
>
> —SIR FRANCIS BACON

Let me now explore the relationship between music and medicine. Shakespeare said:

The man that hath no music in himself,
Nor is not mov'd with concord of sweet sounds,
Is fit for treasons, stratagems, and spoils.

Music to me, and to many, is the greatest of all arts. Great music can induce a state of ecstatic joy, lull one into a state of contemplative, detached serenity, or arouse passions that make the heart tremble with excitement. Music can be the most emotive of arts, followed by poetry, and then perhaps by literature and the visual arts. We hear music with our ears, but the mechanism of its emotive response, or the overall musical experience, is still a mystery that largely remains unsolved.

The history of human civilization reveals that in every culture, from the primitive to the modern, music is an immortal force that allows people to express emotions and to communicate with one another. Other than simply expressing emotions, music can equally alter them. It was the British dramatist William Congreve who wrote in 1697:

> Musick hath Charms to soothe a savage Breast,
> To soften Rocks, or bend a knotted Oak.

Music also has the power to assuage suffering and to confer calm and peace to the troubled mind. Studies have shown that music is helpful to patients; it induces a state of relaxation, can reduce blood pressure, heart rate, stress hormones, pain and the need for pain medication. It can lift depression, eliminate fear and induce positive thoughts, enabling the patient to fight anxiety and depression successfully. It is being increasingly used in cancer patients, where a positive approach induced by listening daily to music or performing it singly or in a group goes a long way in achieving better outcomes. Appropriate music needs to be used for this purpose, for just as some music can soothe or calm, other music can excite and produce undesirable physiological changes within the body. I have tried music therapy in the hospital setting and have advised music therapy to selected patients in my consulting practice. There are some works of music that are indeed particularly effective. When heard in a quiet room, more so in the stillness of the night, when most pain is felt more deeply and when troubles may turn into nightmares, these works help to relieve suffering and calm the mind.

Many physicians would ask if there is any evidence to support many of the uses of music in medicine that I have stated above. Fortunately, there is increasing research on the subject and an increasing body of evidence to this effect. There have been quite a few studies showing definite evidence of reduced stress levels (as manifested by reduced blood pressure readings and fall in heart rate) in patients prior to surgery, during surgery and after surgery when they listened to music. The comparison was with patients who did not listen to music. There are also studies to show that patients hearing music during illness or surgery required much less medication for pain compared to those who did not listen to music.

Music has recently been shown to help preserve balance in the elderly. Those trained to walk and perform various movements in time to music showed better gait and balance compared to those who merely continued their usual activities. This is of importance as poor balance is the most important cause of falls and consequent fractures in elderly individuals who otherwise have no neurological disease. I have had a limited but satisfying experience in the use of music therapy in my practice. Let me give a few examples of the musical works one recommends. I frequently recommend the music of Mozart, in particular his Clarinet Concerto in A Major, his flute concertos, some of his sonatas for the violin and piano, the andante of his Piano Concerto in G Major and much of his chamber music. Each is wonderful to listen to, particularly for an individual with a trained musical ear. Both Mozart's and Bach's music weave a spiritual web and produce a remarkable trance-like effect that assuages suffering. Beethoven's music, his sonatas, the andante movement of his Violin Concerto in D Major and Chopin's nocturnes can act likewise.

It is not just Western classical music that exerts this effect. It can be any form of music, from any part of the world, so long as it is soothing and has a special appeal for the listener. It is important to ask the patient to concentrate deeply on the music that he or she hears, to listen to every note, to shut out noises from the mind and to banish every thought that may arise in the mind's eye, as promptly as possible. The more intense the focus on the music, the greater the effect. For those who appreciate Indian music, I recommend soothing ragas played on the sitar by Ravi Shankar or his daughter Anoushka Shankar, the melodious *shehnai* of Ustad Bismillah Khan, or the rhythmic slow ragas of the santoor played by Pandit

Shivkumar Sharma. Equally great, and to many even greater, are the beautifully melodious, heart-rending qawwalis sung in Urdu or Persian by the Sufis—followers of the mystical Sufi strain of Islam These qawwalis are paeans of devotion and love to the old Sufi saints, to the Prophet Mohammed, but above all to God, music assuredly being the only way to evoke him. Listeners sway, clap and lose themselves in the ecstasy of God.

Listen to this qawwali of Rumi, the Sufi saint, even though the cadence, rhythm and sonority of this verse are lost in the translation from the mellifluous Persian to the English language:

> Prayer clears the mist
> And brings back peace to the soul.
> Every morning, every evening
> Let the heart sing
> *La ilaha il Allah.*
> 'There is no reality but God.'

Music therapy is not new. It was used in the Second World War to help soldiers convalesce from wounds, trauma and surgery. The art and science of Ayurveda was familiar with music as a form of treatment. An ancient Indian study known as Nada yoga acknowledges the effect of different ragas on the mind and body. This has come down to us as the Raga Chikitsa, which is really music therapy. According to the Raga Chikitsa, different ragas are prescribed for different ailments. For example, the Raga Todi is believed to reduce hypertension; Raga Marwa, to relieve fever.

How does music therapy act? How do harmony, rhythm and tempo help to heal? Is music medicine? If so, what is the scientific basis of its action? Although until recently much of the clinical use of music was based on unproven methods, there is today an emerging body of evidence-based music interventions through peer-reviewed scientific experiments. In the April 2013 edition of *Trends in Cognitive Sciences*, Mona Lisa Chanda and Daniel J. Levitin wrote a feature review titled 'The Neurochemistry of Music'. The ensuing discussion is based entirely on the contents of this review. These authors examine the scientific evidence and opine that music influences health through neurochemical changes in the following four domains.

1. Reward, Motivation and Pleasure

Music, as mentioned earlier, can be strongly emotive and people consider the emotional impact combined with its regulation as two of the main reasons for listening to music. Music can result in intrinsic pleasure, or even euphoria, sometimes experienced as a 'thrill'. Cocaine and other similar drugs of abuse, palatable food, humour are noted to yield activation within mesocorticolimbic structures—these are termed the reward centres. It is postulated that music acts by activating the same neuroanatomical and neurochemical systems. Studies using positron emission tomography (PET) were conducted to investigate regional blood flow changes during experienced musical pleasure trial vis-à-vis regional blood flow changes while listening to neutrally rated music. It was observed that strongly emotive music was associated with a significant increase in cerebral blood flow values within structures that comprise the mesocorticolimbic system and which are critical to reward and reinforcement, such as the nucleus accumbens, midbrain, thalamus and the orbitofrontal cortex. MRI studies suggest that musical reward is dependent on dopaminergic neurotransmission within the same network as other reinforcing stimuli.

2. Stress and Arousal

Listening to relaxing music leads to a reduction in stress levels in various clinical situations listed earlier.

A proposed mechanism for the ability of music to reduce stress, regulate arousal and emotions is through the initiation of reflex brainstem responses. Music modulates brainstem responses such as the heart rate, blood pressure, body temperature, skin conductance and muscle tension. These effects are chiefly mediated by tempo—slow music punctuated by pauses cause a decrease in heart rate, blood pressure and respiration. Faster music produces an increase in these parameters.

3. Immune Function

Does music induce healing through its stimulating action on the immune system of the body? Recent published work by Dr Conrad and his colleagues suggest that the physiological response of critically ill individuals exposed to the soothing music of Mozart was characterized by an unexpected jump in the pituitary growth hormone which is known to be crucial in healing. Earlier reports suggest that listening to Mozart's music can lead to an increased activation of brain regions not directly involved in the process of listening. Music may thus act through the neuroendocrine system which is in a way, a neuronal orchestral conductor directing the body's immune system. Music perhaps stimulates the conductor to get the healing process started. Dr Conrad plans further studies on how music can improve a surgeon's performance. Let me quote Dr Conrad on this subject: 'If I don't play music for a couple of days, I cannot feel things as well in surgery. My hands are not as tender with the tissue. They are not so sensitive to the feedback that the tissue gives you.'

4. Social Affiliation

Evidence suggests that social factors play an important role in improving health outcomes. Music and dance foster feelings of social connections, camaraderie and bonding. Many human activities are rhythmic and as Chanda and Levitin say, 'When rhythmic activities are performed by groups of people they tend to become synchronized, reflecting social coordination'. Oxytocin and vasopressin are two neuropeptides known to regulate social behaviour. Only the role of oxytocin has been investigated in relation to music. The role of vasopressin and the relation between the two is unexplained.

Chanda and Levitin conclude that much 'has been discovered about the neuroanatomical basis for music, whereas not much is known about its neurochemical basis'. They believe that 'studies of the neurochemistry of music may be the next great frontier' for researchers in the field of music.

Music—Its Nature and Significance

Does music have a moral significance? The notion that it does, without reference to anything beyond itself, is indeed both pervasive and enduring. The belief that music can profoundly influence human character and shape morality originated with the ancient Greek philosophers—notably Plato and Aristotle. This belief has percolated down the ages to the present. Plato and Aristotle opined that music has certain intrinsic features that prompted spiritual order and harmony within the soul. The Greeks of Plato's day believed that the right type of music when listened to could build character and moral values and promote order and harmony within. Equally, the wrong type of music was harmful and was therefore to be avoided and should be forbidden.

Theon of Smyrna, a Platonist who lived between 115 and 140 CE, left a treatise concerning arithmetic, astronomy and the theory of musical harmony, which he called *Mathematics Useful for Reading Plato*, in which he says:

The Pythagoreans, whom Plato follows in many respects, call music the harmonization of opposites, the unification of

disparate things and the reconciliation of warring elements…
Music, as they say, is the basis of agreement among things
in nature and of the best government in the universe. As a
rule it assumes the guise of harmony in the universe, of lawful
government in a state, and of a sensible way of life in the
home. It brings together and unites.

I would consider the music one hears in the world today
as great, good, neutral (indifferent) and bad. Great music,
with its emotive power expressed in many ways, ennobles
the listener. Good music is pleasant, relaxing, enlivening,
nostalgic—it makes one forget the worries of life and living.
Neutral music is music to which one is at best indifferent. Bad
music is music that repels one, hurts and harms one. Let me
give just one example of bad music. It is music that consists
of a raucous cacophony of disjointed sounds, deafening to the
ears, lacking both harmony and rhythm; through the music
one often hears a harsh voice, and when one listens with
difficulty to the words, we hear the utterance of incoherent
sentences filled with vulgarity and profanity. Music such as
this is popular with many young people in the West. Surely,
this is music that harms and not heals! Mercifully Indian
music, baring rare exceptions, is free of this taint.

Many would consider the views of Plato and Aristotle
outdated. They mention that the history of the world is a
chronicle of change and that this holds for both the arts and
sciences. Just as the old ideas of the physical world we live
in have been replaced and superseded by the discoveries of
scientists like Copernicus, Galileo, Newton, Leibniz, Einstein,
Plank, Hawkins and several others, old art must give way to
new. But this is not so—art differs from science. In music for
example great music of the past remains great today. The music
of Bach has not been displaced by that of Mozart nor has that
of Mozart been displaced by Beethoven, nor that of Beethoven
supplanted by Rachmaninov or Shostakovich. Great works of

modern music refine our senses and sensibilities, but they do not replace or supplant the great music that preceded them. Why and how is it that music—an art which preaches no doctrine, an art unrelated to the external world, an art dissociated from verbal language and meaning has become so intrinsically woven into the fabric of human thought and the human psyche? Perhaps because it mirrors the inner flow of life. The philosopher Hegel conceived music to be akin to the inner life of human beings, which is pictured as a consciously flowing stream. Philosopher Henri Bergson echoes this concept when he refers to 'the continuous melody of our inner life—a melody which is going on and will go on, indivisible, from the beginning to the end of our conscious existence'. The musical theorist Heinrich Schenker writes, 'In its linear progression and comparable tonal events, music mirrors the human soul in all its metamorphoses and moods'.

Music is related to the visual arts, literature and poetry because each has an aesthetic beauty. It is also unrelated in that it cannot be seen, is comprehended but cannot be translated, and it bears no relation to the external world. Amazingly music seems to have a fair degree of similarity with mathematics. Music is characterized by the beauty of tones; mathematicians speak of the beauty of numbers. Both are concerned with the linking together of abstractions and making patterns of ideas. Ludwig Wittgenstein, a philosopher who loved and felt music deeply, spoke of the great beauty of Bertrand Russell's, *Principia Mathematica* and said what was probably the greatest praise he could give it—that it was like music. A. J. Whitehead in his Lowell lectures of 1925 spoke thus—'The science of Pure Mathematics, in its modern developments, may claim to be the most original creation of the human spirit. Another claimant for the position is music'.

My interest in the mathematician Hardy stems from his association in Cambridge with the Indian mathematical genius Srinivasa Ramanujan. My interest was intensified when I discovered his views on mathematics were closely similar to those of many discerning musicians on great music. Hardy opined that pure mathematics was independent of the physical world, and a mathematical concept was not concerned with any practical application it might have in the future. He observed that serious mathematical ideas are characterized by generality, depth, inevitability, economy and unexpectedness. Amazingly, these are the very characteristics of both great Western and great Indian classical music. Great music must have a general appeal; it is neither bound by nor does it respect frontiers; it is not restricted to a national idiom or a national ethos. It must have substance, depth; a lack of depth signifies monotony and commonplace rhythm as we see in popular music today. Perhaps, most important of all, it is characterized by inevitability. This indeed is a feature of all great art. When complete it gives one the feeling it could never have been composed any other way. There is one difference between the inevitability of mathematical ideas and great music, or for that matter other great art forms. The progress of great music to its eventual climax and conclusion is *aesthetically* inevitable, while the progress of mathematical ideas towards their conclusion is *logically* inevitable.

Unexpectedness is one other feature; it is characterized by the construction of new patterns, and unexpected tones and harmony. Unexpectedness is linked to inevitability and in a way to originality, leaving the listener with the feeling that the music could not have been other than what it is. Economy is important but perhaps not as important as the other characteristics. It does not always apply to great music. For example, the works of Wagner are opulent in duration; a concise, economical Wagnerian composition that is truly great is inconceivable. In general, as Storr says, 'the indivisibility of form and content powerfully contributes to our feeling of inevitability'.

If the qualities that characterize pure mathematics as expounded by famous mathematicians are similar to those in great music, where lies the difference? I feel it is the unique and beautiful combination of mathematics and magic that makes music different, giving music a special mystique. Its magic rests in its evocative powers—both intellectual and emotional, and in its ability through these evocative powers to mirror all aspects of life. In rare moments, its magic conveys what Freud described Romain Rolland as calling 'a sensation of "eternity," a feeling of something limitless, unbounded—as it were "oceanic"'. It's a feeling in which the listener merges as one with the universe around him. Above all, great music reveals the inherent spirituality with which humans are endowed, prompting them to seek and realize their true selves, which is the ultimate goal of life on earth.

We must finally ask a rather pertinent question. Are the 'patterns' of mathematics and music human inventions or 'are they discoveries of a pre-existing order'. Amazingly, Hardy who was a diehard atheist believed that mathematical theorems are not so much creations as observations or discoveries. Sir Roger Penrose agrees with this view. He asks, 'Are mathematicians really uncovering truths which are, in fact, already there—truths whose existence is quite independent of the mathematicians' activities?' However, in my opinion, great music cannot and does not have an independent existence. It is the creation and the priceless product of great minds revealing everlasting truths. It is only when the composer can reach down into the hidden depths of his or her psyche, draw forth hidden emotions from buried experiences to a conscious level and impart to them the ordered structure of sound, that great music is born.

I believe it is feeling rather than intellect that enables an artist, a composer, to transform experience, transcend reality so as to reach a point beyond it. What enables a great composer to do so? This is a question that has no answer. It is a gift either inborn or acquired that enables him or her to do so; an attempt to describe the genesis of this gift would be an exercise in futility. At times, this gift amounts to real genius, as in the case of Wolfgang Amadeus Mozart who started composing at the age of six years when experience, hidden or overt, hardly mattered. This inner ordering process described above is largely unconscious and not deliberated or willed by the composer. Aristotle called this phenomenon 'inspiration'. It is a process for which the composer waits often in unmitigated agony until like a flash of lightning it is suddenly and often unexpectedly realized. Amazingly, it is often the troubled mind, a mind agonised by physical or mental suffering, that is blessed with an inspirational force. The great creative achievements in the history of the world emanate from the human brain, yet it does not necessarily follow that they are entirely voluntary constructs. The brain is the most mysterious of all organs; it may well function in mysterious ways that are not necessarily under voluntary control.

Finally, how does one distinguish great music and other great works of art from lesser works? I can do no better than quote Penrose for an answer:

> Great works of art are indeed 'closer to God' than are lesser ones. It is a feeling not uncommon among artists, that in their greatest works they are revealing eternal truths which have some kind of prior ethereal existence, while their lesser works might be more arbitrary, of the nature of mere mortal constructions.

I have often wondered when listening to great music, be it Western or Indian, what does it all mean, what is its purpose, its significance? Music makes me believe that there is a world beyond the world we inhabit, that the *spirit*, the *self*, within us is birthless, deathless, infinite. Music allows us to commune with our inner stream of consciousness and with the supreme being. In doing so, music gives meaning to life, a transcendental blessing that enriches, enhances and ennobles the human spirit.

8

Medicine in the Renaissance Era

Je le pansai, Dieu le guérit.
[I dressed him, God healed him.]

—AMBROISE PARÉ

The fall of Rome and the disintegration of the western part of the Roman Empire ushered in the Dark Ages, an era during which there was an eclipse in the civilization of the West. More generally, this era includes the period between 470 and 1000 CE. Many historians of today find the value judgement implicit in the term 'Dark Ages' unacceptable and prefer not to use it. Yet, it is an incontrovertible fact that this period of history in the West was marked by strife, disorder, chaos, pestilence and war, intellectual darkness and barbarity. The Dark Ages began to see the light of day around 1000 CE, but it was only with the birth of the Renaissance in the fourteenth century that darkness was dispelled and the sun shone in full splendour over the Western world.

The Renaissance (derived from the Italian term '*la rinascita*', meaning 'rebirth') was an Italian phenomenon born and centred in Italy, but like a gentle breeze, its influence spread through the rest of western and northern Europe. The essence of the Renaissance was the concept of humanism. Humanism constituted a total change in the outlook on life when compared to the Middle Ages. Most importantly, it broke dogmas that were handed down from the past and searched for truth and knowledge, preferred philosophy to religion, studied nature, glorified the individual, and in the words of poet Alexander Pope, believed—'The proper study of mankind is man'. The true Renaissance man was a multifaceted personality who could embrace with equal aptitude literature, philosophy, architecture, astronomy and medicine. Yet, at the same time, he was proficient in fencing, hunting, music, dancing, and in the courtly arts.

Yet, we must remind ourselves that the Renaissance era was not just heaven on earth, nor just an era of peace and plenty, or of happiness and virtue. Unbridled individualism, besides exerting a liberating influence on the thoughts of mankind, also bred tyranny, passion and violence. In fact, this was a period of incredible contrasts—richness and splendour of the mind contrasted with despicable treachery; nobility of the spirit, with a decadent moral code; beneficence, with cruelty. Nevertheless, when we look back in history and contemplate this era, the violence and the cruelty fall into the shadows and the splendour and glory of its achievements rise before our eyes like a breathtaking vision—the vision of being lost forever in a sun-drenched beautiful garden.

Medicine and Humanism

Physicians of this era were predominantly humanists. The accomplished Renaissance physician was primarily a man of letters, equally learned in arts, philosophy and literature, as in medicine. Physicians generally belonged to a wealthier class, educated as they were in the famous universities of Padua, Bologna and Ferrara in Italy. Padua, particularly, attracted a number of foreign students from all over Europe. The constitution of almost every university in Italy vested great powers in the student community. It was the student body that elected the officials and debated and decided on the curriculum of studies. In the true spirit of the Renaissance, the universities became increasingly secular, freeing themselves from religious dogma and ecclesiastical control.

Let me give some examples of great humanist physicians who combined the study and practice of medicine with other human endeavours. Niccolò Leoniceno (1428–1524) was famous for his vitriolic attack on the Galenic doctrine. He is also the author of one of the earliest medical texts on syphilis. He undertook the correction of botanical errors in Pliny's *Natural History* and founded a medical school in Ferrara, where he was an outstanding clinician. Geronimo Cardano (1501–76) was a physician, mathematician, astrologer, musician, and the author of a great Renaissance autobiography *De vita propria liber* (The book of my life). His treatise titled *De malo recentiorum medicorum mendendi usu* (The bad practice of healing among modern doctors) was a scathing indictment of the practice of doctors in this era, earning him opprobrium and scorn from his fellow physicians. His work was the forerunner by over four hundred years of Ivan Illich's *Medical Nemesis: The Expropriation of Health* (1975). Thomas Linacre (*ca.* 1460–1524) was a humanist and physician who established chairs in philosophy at Oxford and Cambridge and who founded the Royal College of Physicians of London. He was physician to Henry VIII and to Cardinal Wolsey and a great friend of Desiderius Erasmus, one of the great humanist scholars of that age.

Another great humanist scholar of this age was Nicolaus Copernicus (1473–1543) He was Polish and was an accomplished mathematician, astronomer, theologian and physician. He studied theology in Bologna and medicine in Padua. He practised medicine at Frauenberg in East Prussia and at the same time discharged his religious duties as canon of the town cathedral. His accomplishments in mathematics, theology, and as a physician are forgotten, but he achieved immortality after the publication of *De revolutionibus orbium coelestium* (On the revolutions of the heavenly spheres). He received on his deathbed the first printed copy of his work, which demolished the Ptolemaic theory that the earth was the centre of universe. He wrote that it was the earth that moved around the sun. He died a happy and fulfilled man.

Girolamo Fracastoro

Smallpox, plague, malaria, typhoid and other waterborne infections occurred sporadically as also in epidemic form—a legacy to mankind since civilization began. Scurvy was epidemic in sailors at sea; rickets was a common affliction of children in this era.

A new devastating disease, occurring in epidemic form, characterized by fever, rash, severe prostration with circulatory collapse and death, was accurately described by Girolamo Fracastoro (*ca.* 1478–1553). This scourge was typhus and assumed an epidemic form when human beings were crowded together in unsanitary conditions in the cold of winter. The Spanish army suffered severely from typhus during the siege of Granada, losing over seventeen thousand soldiers. In 1529, typhus nearly decimated a French army besieging Naples.

Girolamo Fracastoro was one of the greatest humanists who adorned the Renaissance. Fracastoro was a wealthy Veronese gentleman who studied with his fellow student Copernicus in the University of Padua in the early sixteenth century. He then lived as a country squire and a practising physician on his country estate in Verona. He was also a poet, a playwright, and was known to carry a book of classics to read as he made his leisurely medical rounds precariously perched on the back of a mule. After practising medicine for twenty years, he took solely to literary pursuits.

Fracastoro wrote poetry, plays, and also treatises on literature, geography and astronomy. He wrote two major medical works. The 'love sickness' or rather the 'love pestilence' excited his interest as a poet, a physician and an epidemiologist. His poem *Syphilis sive morbus Gallicus* (Syphilis or the French disease) ran into three volumes and was published in 1525 and 1530. It was written in Latin and described the origin, clinical features and treatment of this disease. Many consider it to be the most widely known poem in medical literature. Fracastoro's second and greater contribution was his treatise titled *De contagione et contagiosis morbis* (On contagion and contagious diseases) published in 1546. This book postulated the principles related to the cause and spread of underlying contagious diseases. He suggested that invisible germs called '*seminaria*' caused contagious diseases and he stressed the need to destroy these seminaria. He described three forms of contagion—direct contact; indirect contact by way of clothing, linen, personal belongings and utensils; and finally, contact through distance propagated by germs in the air. This Renaissance man was the first to give an excellent description of typhus in medicine and differentiate it from plague. He also emphasized the infectious nature of tuberculosis, which was a common affliction in Europe.

Indeed Fracastoro was a great humanist, who contributed not only to medicine but also to the beginnings of epidemiology and to several other human endeavours. The seminaria that he postulated as being responsible for the cause and spread of infectious diseases anticipated the germ theory of infection postulated and proved by Louis Pasteur nearly three hundred years later.

The Story of Syphilis and of Girolamo Fracastoro

The 'great pox' later named syphilis made its dramatic entry in the Renaissance era. This dreadful disease was a scourge on par with plague and smallpox. It was observed in the soldiers of Charles VIII of France during the siege of Naples in 1493. It was then termed *'mal Napolitain'* (the Neapolitan disease). Naples surrendered without a fight, but the disbanded soldiers, mercenaries and their camp followers spread the disease all over Europe. The disease was characterized by disfiguring sores and ulcers on the skin and a repulsive rash. The disease was called by various names. The Italians as an insult to the French called it *mal Francese*. Other terms were *'morbus Gallicus'*, *'morbo Lusitano'* and *'mal Spagnole'*; the term in general use was morbus Gallicus.

The story of syphilis is worth recounting. In 1530, Girolamo Fracastoro published the previously mentioned poem *Syphilis sive morbus Gallicus*. In this poem, a shepherd named Syphilis insults the Greek god Apollo. Apollo seeks revenge by striking the shepherd with a scourge, which causes the flesh from his limbs to decay and fall, revealing his bones; his teeth fall out, his breath becomes foetid and his voice is reduced to a whisper. The great pox now universally became known as 'syphilis'.

It is even now a commonly held belief that syphilis was introduced to Europe and from Europe to the world at large from America through Columbus's sailors. A Seville physician Ruy Diaz de Isla, who treated these sailors, was of the opinion that the sailors contracted the disease during their halt in Haiti. Yet, there is evidence that the disease existed well before Columbus discovered America. A typical syphilitic crural ulcer has been depicted in a 1461 painting, and medieval medical manuscripts describe cases of venereal leprosy that may well have been cutaneous syphilis. Fracastoro noted that the disease occurred simultaneously in many countries and cast doubt on the fact that Columbus' sailors introduced it into Europe. It is likely that the *Treponema pallidum* (the spirochaete causing syphilis that was discovered over three centuries later) existed in the Old World before the discovery of America. Perhaps in the fifteenth century, the organism underwent a mutation, thereby making it extremely invasive in hosts (both in Europe and America) who till then were resistant to the organism. There might be a close analogy between the outbreak of syphilis in the fifteenth century and the spread of HIV infection in the late twentieth century. The notion that syphilis was brought by Columbus's sailors from America could well have been driven by commercial interests. Guaiacum or guaiac, 'the holy wood', was being used by the natives of America and was brought by Spanish sailors to Europe as an effective therapy for syphilis. Even Fracastoro was enthusiastic over the guaiac treatment for syphilis, though it was later proved to be useless. Trading companies in the Baltic controlled the import of guaiac from America, and belief in the worth of this 'New World cure' was perpetuated by this trade.

Within a few decades of its description, it was established that syphilis was related and spread by sexual contact. Doctors in Scotland were the first to realize this and threatened to brand women as being of ill fame if they continued to work as prostitutes. The enigma of this horrific disease was now solved, for conditions in Europe were ideally conducive to its sexual spread. Rome earned over thirty thousand scudi a year from taxes levied on the brothels in the city. Venice with a population of three hundred thousand had twelve thousand prostitutes. Prostitution and a hedonistic code of living fuelled the spread of syphilis far and wide. There was a campaign against prostitution and prostitutes. Some countries banned prostitution and prostitutes; some made the examination of prostitutes compulsory. Special hospitals were established to treat the 'great pox', and at some of these, the community provided free treatment. Besides the use of guaiac as a treatment for syphilis, the only treatment available was the application of mercury as an ointment. The 'greasers of pox', who were often quacks rather than physicians, smeared the whole body with the 'Saracenic ointment' promising cure. 'A night with Venus and a lifetime with Mercury', was the quip often used by those unscarred by the disease. Bloodletting, purging and hot baths were the age-old methods used to eliminate the 'syphilitic vapour' from the body—all to no avail.

The Great Renaissance Rebels in Medicine

The Renaissance inherited the Galenic doctrines in medicine. Galen was a great physician who lived and worked in the second century CE. He undoubtedly made great contributions in anatomy, physiology and clinical diagnosis. But, great as he was, he made many mistakes as many men do. The tragedy of his mistakes is unique in that they were perpetuated for over fifteen hundred years after his death. There must be indeed few mistakes in the history of human endeavour that would equal this unenviable record. All that Galen wrote about medicine was considered to be gospel truth that could not be questioned; anyone who did so was considered a heretic and ostracized. Galen could think and write no wrong! This attitude, as mentioned before, stood for fifteen hundred years after his death. Medicine stood frozen, fossilized, during this period.

The Renaissance produced humanists that blazed a great trail of splendour and beauty in painting and sculpture, literature and philosophy. Medicine unfortunately lagged far behind. There was nothing in the Renaissance to match for example the brilliant discovery of the circulation by William Harvey in the seventeenth century, no breakthrough in diagnosis or treatment, no drug of sufficient merit to counter suffering and disease. It was difficult to break the shackles of Galenic doctrines and theories. However, then strode on to the Renaissance stage three great rebels in medicine, each bold enough to sound on his own the death knell of Galenism and change the path of medicine from dogma and doctrine to that of true scientific inquiry. They were Andreas Vesalius (1514–64), the anatomist; Paracelsus (1493–1541), the physician; and Ambroise Paré (1510–90), the surgeon. There was a fourth individual, Leonardo da Vinci (1452–1519), the like of whom the world has yet to produce, a quintessential Renaissance man, who in addition to his numerous contributions to almost every field of human endeavour, made great contributions to the science of anatomy. I need to give you a brief description of each of these heroes who epitomized the advance of medicine in this era.

ANDREAS VESALIUS

Andreas Vesalius is renowned and celebrated the world over as the 'father of modern anatomy'. Born in Brussels in 1514, he was of Flemish descent. His magnum opus *De humani corporis fabrica libri septem* (seven books on the structure of the human anatomy) published in 1543, when he was just twenty-eight years old, is one of the greatest books in medical science.

Vesalius came from a family of distinguished physicians, his father being the apothecary to Charles V. Vesalius first studied at Louvain and then at the University of Montpellier and University of Paris successively. When at the University of Paris, he and his fellow students were known to raid the cemeteries and bring back corpses for dissection at home. In 1537, Vesalius went to the University of Padua and graduated with distinction in medicine in one year. Remarkably, the day after he received his university degree, he was appointed professor of anatomy. The very next day after this appointment, he commenced his dissection work, and his lectures and discourses on human anatomy were often given while dissecting dead bodies. His brilliance attracted students and scholars from all over Europe. After five years of brilliant dissection, experimentation and observation, Vesalius discarded the old Galenic dogmas of anatomy and published the previously mentioned magnum opus *De humani corporis fabrica libri septem.* In 1543, Vesalius introduced the concept of 'living' anatomy. Vesalius drew the anatomical concept in the living position with the help of his fellow contemporary Jan van Calcar and perhaps also with the help of Titian and other artists of the Titian school. The Padua landscape was an artistic background to his anatomical sketches. The sketches were engraved on wood, and three hundred printing blocks of these engravings were sent on mule back across the Alps to the master printer Johannes Oporinus. This monumental work was written by a man not yet thirty years old. Galenic myths, which had been left untouched and uncorrected for over a thousand years, were now shattered— he is known to have corrected two hundred Galenic errors. In doing so, he demolished hallowed concepts in medicine that had well-nigh become religious beliefs.

The shock to the world of medicine was profound. How could a man just twenty-eight years old dare to challenge and correct Galenic doctrines on anatomy which had stood as gospel truth for fifteen hundred years? Like many great discoverers, he was ridiculed and hounded by his fellow colleagues and accused by the church and clergy of heresy for refuting many of the truths of the Galenic doctrines. Unable to withstand the torments hurled at him, Vesalius burnt all his remaining unpublished manuscripts and fled from Padua to become physician to Charles V and then to Philip III of Spain. In 1563, he journeyed on a pilgrimage to Jerusalem. On his return, his ship was wrecked on the island of Zante in the Ionian Sea. He died on this island, probably of typhoid, in 1564. Thus was destroyed a great man in the very prime of his life by the bigotry, jealousy and hate of the lesser mortals of our world.

PARACELSUS

Paracelsus was the rebel physician of the Renaissance who fearlessly declaimed the dogmas and doctrines prevalent in medicine. His real name was Philippus Aureolus Theophrastus Bombastus von Hohenheim. A sworn enemy of bigotry and tradition, he named himself Paracelsus, suggesting that he was even greater than Celsus, who practised and wrote on medicine in the early years of the Christian era. Paracelsus was of Teutonic descent and was born in 1493 in Switzerland. His father was a doctor who left Switzerland for Austria, and the young Theophrastus was introduced to the mysteries of alchemy and astrology by the abbot of the monastery at Würzberg. He then briefly studied at Vienna, Paris, Montpellier, and finally took his medical degree in Ferrara in 1519.

Paracelsus was an iconoclast who set out on his peripatetic travels. His writings suggest that he must have visited Poland, Russia, Lithuania, Spain and the greater part of Western Europe. He communed with the common people and wrote, 'I have not been ashamed to learn from tramps, butchers and barbers things which seemed of use to me'. Though brilliant, his ideas were often couched in obscure language. His writings were a potpourri of medicine, natural science, religion, astrology, magic and alchemy. He was a classic example of a strongly opinionated man of the Renaissance who combined humanity with intolerance. Rather coarse in his behaviour and fond of drink, he made many enemies and alienated many friends.

He was a strong opponent of Galen, yet erred in postulating that all matter was composed from sulphur, mercury and salt. His peripatetic travels ceased when he was asked to treat the

Basle humanist and master publisher Johannes Frobenius in 1526. Frobenius had an inflamed leg and was advised amputation to save his life by several physicians. Paracelsus treated and cured him. Soon after, the great Erasmus described his own illness in a letter to Paracelsus. Paracelsus again cured him. These two incidents catapulted him to fame, and he was offered a university chair in Basle—a far cry from his earlier wandering existence among the meek and the lowly. Even so, Paracelsus remained true to his self. His first speech as a university professor was delivered in German instead of the customary Latin. He followed this break in tradition by publicly burning the works of Galen and Avicenna, a heresy that many never forgave him. He also publicly denounced his colleagues for propagating dogma and falsehood instead of searching for the truth. He kept his post in Basle for two years, which were dogged by controversy and dispute. He finally resigned and reverted to his vagabond existence, dying in 1541 at Salzburg at the age of forty-two years.

In spite of his failings and his egoistic arrogance, Paracelsus was a great Renaissance man. He broke the shackles that bound medicine to wrong traditions, dogma and false beliefs, and he pointed to the path that should be followed. He himself did not take more than a few steps on this path, but opened the way for future generations to follow. He must have been a great physician of his time and age, for he looked at medicine with fresh eyes.

AMBROISE PARÉ

Ambroise Paré was the most famous and renowned surgeon of the Renaissance and one of the greatest surgeons of all time. His life story is fascinating and illustrates how surgery broke new grounds during this era.

In 1536, Francis, King of France, cast his covetous eyes on rich Turin and on the Duchy of Savoy in Northern Italy. He marched his troops into Piedmont attacking the forts guarding that area. The carnage was horrific, and the battlefields were strewn with the dead and the wounded. The wounds were chiefly gunshot wounds, and the surgeons in the French army had a lot of work on their hands. Ambrois Paré was a young barber-surgeon who had joined the service of Francis, King of France. This was his first experience of war, and his baptism into surgery was indeed by fire. He had never seen gunshot wounds before, but was taught that gunshot wounds were poisonous because of the gunpowder within them and that the treatment of such wounds consisted of cauterizing them with burning oil of elder mixed with treacle. Realizing the agony that this would cause to the wounded, he asked the senior surgeons as to what they used for their initial dressing. He was told to pour burning oil into the wounds. Paré did this with great trepidation. Fortunately, both for him and his wounded patients, he ran short of oil. Perhaps a lesser person would have gone in search for more oil or retired to a campfire to escape the horrors of the battlefield. Paré, through intuition, innovation, or through sheer chance (we shall never know), began to apply a mixture of egg yolk, oil of roses and turpentine to the wounds. On awakening at the break of dawn, he was astonished to find those on whom he had used his mixture felt little pain, and their wounds were not inflamed, while those who had been cauterized with burning oil were in great pain, and their wounds were markedly inflamed. He vowed never to use burning oil on gunshot wounds. A mere novice of a barber-surgeon thus exorcised forever the cruel practice of scorching wounds with burning oil or with a red-hot iron.

Unlike most humanist physicians, barber-surgeons lacked education, were ignorant in Latin, were impecunious, and were unable to enter universities. Paré was born in Bourg-Hesent in the department of Mayenne in 1510. His father and uncle were both barber-surgeons. Unable to go to a university he learnt his art and craft as an apprentice to a relative barber-surgeon and then as a resident surgeon at the Hôtel-Dieu in Paris—an old hospital founded by monks in the Middle Ages. As an army surgeon his young mind had not been prejudiced by the teachings of earlier centuries. He had no reverence for Galen and those that succeeded Galen. In his treatise on gunshot wounds, written in French, he wrote 'I do not wish to be able to boast to have read Galen in the Greek or in the Latin; God was not pleased to be so kind to me in my youth so as to provide for instruction in the one or the other of these languages'. He taught himself, learning from observation, experience and experiment. He was compassionate, considerate, innovative and, above all, singularly modest for a surgeon of such brilliance. In his first encounter with death and suffering, during the French Piedmont campaign, a badly wounded officer named Le Rat was brought to him. The young barber saved his life and when asked how, made the historic remark: '*Je le pansai, Dieu le guérit*' (I dressed him, God healed him). This is the remark that has been engraved on his tombstone. It was indeed a profound remark—an expression of his innate humility and devoutness, of faith and trust in God and in the healing power of nature.

Ambroise Paré wrote extensively in his diaries on what he saw and did. The illness of Marquis d'Auret detailed below, illustrates not only his approach to diagnosis and management but also his faith in the healing power of nature and his close communion with a very sick man—factors that promoted healing and recovery in what seemed a mortal illness.

Marquis d'Auret had his femur shattered by a gunshot wound and in spite of being treated for several months by several doctors was at death's door. The king of France requested Paré to treat him. Paré describes beautifully the clinical features of infection and sepsis: 'I found him in a high fever, his eyes deep sunken, …his tongue dry and parched, and the whole body much wasted and lean, the voice low as of a man very near death'. Paré found a deep, filthy suppurating wound with bone fragments embedded within. The patient had extensive bedsores, got no rest by day or by night, and was close to death. His sheets were incredibly dirty, stained, and had not been changed for months for the fear of causing pain to the patient. Paré writes, 'It seemed to me there was little hope he would escape death. All the same, to give him courage and good hope, I told him I would soon set him on his legs, by the grace of God, and the help of his physicians and surgeons'. Paré incised and drained the suppurating wound, removed the bone fragments embedded within, ordered a good bath, a clean bed, and positioned d'Auret skilfully to relieve both pressure and discomfort from his bedsores. Paré devised a device whereby drops of water falling into a basin made a sound like rain, thereby lulling the patient to sleep and allowing him the rest he had been badly denied so long. He also ensured that the gloom in the household was replaced by good cheer and by song and sweet music. Marquis d'Auret recovered and lived to write his tale.

I have on purpose described the above illness in detail as it illustrates that medicine and surgery constitute both an art and a science and that the art of medicine consists of the art of healing not just treating, not even curing. Paré illustrated this beautifully when the science of medicine was in its infancy. Modern physicians unfortunately often fail to realize this at a point in time when the science of medicine and surgery are far more advanced.

Ambroise Paré is credited with a number of great discoveries and innovations. I would be failing in my duty to a great man if I did not briefly mention them. He devised, among other surgical instruments, the haemostatic forceps and practised vascular ligation of the arteries to arrest haemorrhage. He improved upon several operative techniques, was a pioneer and founder of modern obstetrics, and the first to put into successful practice podalic version to correct abnormal foetal positions.

Paré lived through the wars of the Reformation initiated by Calvin and Luther. Some historians considered him a Huguenot, but this is unlikely. Whatever be his faith, he was a Christian at heart, with Christian motives and practising Christian charity. He was brave enough to treat the leader of the Huguenots, Admiral Coligny. This was considered a mortal sin at the time of the massacre of St Bartholomew. His life was spared only through the intervention of the king of France.

Destiny beckoned and rewarded this humble barber-surgeon with worldly glory. He became councillor of state and surgeon to four kings of France—Henry II, Frances II, Charles IX and Henry III. He died in 1590, revered as a great surgeon and a great man. Ah, would to God that more surgeons were cast in his mould! He was the scintillating star of the Renaissance whose light shines through centuries to the present day.

LEONARDO DA VINCI—THE RENAISSANCE MAN

The greatest man of the Renaissance and perhaps the greatest man of all time was Leonardo da Vinci. Let me first describe his prowess in anatomy, as this science is an indispensable and important aspect of medicine. Da Vinci studied anatomy by dissecting thirty dead bodies by candlelight in the sanctuary of Santo Spirito. He was then in the service of the Borgia family in Rome. He placed no reliance on what other anatomists wrote or believed. He was meticulous in his observations and wrote down what he saw during his dissections. Of the 6,000 closely written pages in his diary, 190 pages are devoted to anatomy. He left 750 illustrative anatomical drawings, of which 50 illustrated the structure of the heart. He described the auricles but did not grasp the significance of the septum separating the right ventricle from the left. Had he done so,

206 Tabiyat: Medicine and Healing in India and Other Essays

he might well have discovered circulation. He made superb drawings to illustrate what he saw—the coronary arteries and several other anatomical structures. He analysed the muscular system to perfection—the origin of each muscle, its insertion, and its action; he illustrated this through copious notes and superb drawings. It appears from his drawings and notes that he planned a major treatise on anatomy in conjunction with Marcantonio della Torre of Verona. This was not to be because of the premature death of della Torre. Leonardo da Vinci was recognized in his lifetime, and forever, as an artist, sculptor, inventor, engineer, scientist and philosopher. He would almost certainly rank with Andreas Vesalius as the father of modern anatomy if his notebook had not remained undiscovered for two centuries.

I need to digress a bit from the beaten path of medicine to which da Vinci made a worthy contribution. How would one consider da Vinci in the history of Man? He was unquestionably a genius of unsurpassed versatility. Perhaps it required a background of Renaissance thought and Renaissance beliefs and way of life that produced a man of great distinction. As with many great men, he had no preformed concepts of ancient learning or wisdom; he only believed what he saw, found, and discovered through meticulous study and experiments. It is almost incredible that he combined within himself the excellence of all arts and all science. Yet he did!

As an artist and a painter, he had a thirst to unravel the secrets of human anatomy; to learn the laws of proportion and perspective; to study the composition, reflection, and absorption of light; and to study the chemistry of oils and paints used in his canvases. The artist within him brought out the scientist so that art and science mingled and reinforced each other to form a single unit.

Which one of us possess the knowledge and talent in science and art to gauge such a multifaceted personality? One could argue that Titian and Rafael left greater treasures of painting, that Michelangelo was a superior sculptor, or that there were superior engineers, scientists and philosophers. Yet, da Vinci was the man who was all these together and rivalled the best in each field. No canvas of Rafael, Titian, or Michelangelo could match the beautiful composition, poignant thought and feeling of da Vinci's *The Last Supper* or surpass the beautiful lines of *The Virgin and the Child with St Anne*. No philosopher of the Renaissance times could compare with da Vinci's conception of natural laws.

Leonardo da Vinci died at the age of sixty-four on 2 May 1519. A friend who witnessed his death wrote—'The loss of such a man is mourned by all, for it is not in the power of nature to create another.'

The Renaissance Ends

Just as the sun rises, it also sets. It set over the Renaissance towards the end of the sixteenth century and a new age was born—the Baroque Period. This is in the order of things, for the march of history is a chronicle of change. Yet, through the mists of past centuries, we can picture Vesalius exploding Galenic myths and visualize his triumphant smile on the frontispiece of his great treatise; still gaze with rapture on the smile of Mona Lisa wondering how mankind could have produced so multifaceted a man as Leonardo Da Vinci who singly adorned every field of human endeavour. We think back on many other distinguished individuals in this remarkable age who gave nobility to thought and held forth a light to our world that has remained undimmed for centuries.

9

Death

It is not death I fear to face but dying.

—ROBERT LOUIS STEVENSON

Death has been a subject of discussion through the ages. Authors, poets, philosophers, teachers and prophets of so many different religions have expounded on its manifold aspects. Who really knows and speaks the truth? Death mocks them all, for no traveller who has passed beyond the frontier of life to enter the domain of death has ever returned to tell the tale.

It is believed that since humans are at the very top of the evolutionary ladder of living beings, they are the only animals who know that they must die. When and how does a human being learn the certainty of death? Is it an inborn aspect of human life or is it, as Voltaire believes, learnt as a matter of experience. Let me quote Voltaire's view on this: 'The human race is the only one that knows it must die, and it knows this only through its experience. A child brought up alone and transported to a desert island would have no more idea of death than a cat or plant.'

But how does Voltaire, or any individual, assume that an animal is not aware of death, does not have an inborn instinct of its eventual demise, or does not learn from experience that death is a certainty? There are some who feel that consciousness is an attribute restricted to humans, while others feel that all living beings have 'consciousness'. Perhaps the attribute of consciousness is associated with the instinct of eventual death. This is, of course, a surmise, a conjecture, bringing into focus the fact that the certainty of death remains covered by a cloud of uncertainty with regard to what immediately precedes or follows the event.

Having practised the art and science of medicine for several years, I have often asked myself—can one attempt to define death? One must to start with the assertion that if there were no life there would be no death. Also, the moment we are born, we live in the shadow of death. This is elegantly summarized by Francis Quarles when he writes—'He that begins to live begins to die'. Let me quote the quatrain that contains this line in full:

Forbear, fond taper: what thou seek'st, is fire:
Thy own destruction's lodg'd in thy desire;
Thy wants are far more safe than their supply:
He that begins to live begins to die.

Julian of Norwich, a fourteenth-century English mystic, wrote, 'We wot that our parents do but bear us into death. A strange thing, that'. In the book *The Upanishads: The Classics of Indian Spirituality* (1987), Eknath Easwaran interprets these lines as thus:

Birth is but the beginning of a trajectory to death; for all their love, parents cannot halt it and in a sense have 'given us to death', merely by giving us birth!

One often wonders, does life precede death or does death precede life? In his essay 'Beyond the Pleasure Principle', Freud believes that when the universe was born, life was non-existent. Therefore death, in the form of non-existence, preceded life, and evolution has been a continuous struggle into 'back-sliding into the status quo ante'. Life is the distance between the point of birth and the point of death; the distance may be short or long, straight or circuitous; each one charts his or her own course, his or her own path to death.

Donne likens death 'to a translation into a better language—an accession into the great library of eternity', and Saint Francis of Assisi blesses God 'for our sister, the death of the body'. Admittedly, all that I have written does not actually define death; words of poets, authors, philosophers and scientists also merely skirt the issue and do not define it.

There is a view held by some poets and philosophers that when we die, we do not exist, so death does not exist for us. Hence, should the subject of death really exist and should it be flogged endlessly as has been done through the ages? In one of his letters to Menoeceus, the philosopher Epicurus wrote:

So death, the most terrifying of ills, is nothing to us, since so long as we exist, death is not with us; but when death comes, then we do not exist. It does not then concern either the living or the dead, since for the former it is not, and the latter are no more.

The sages in the East (as expressed in the Upanishads) hold that death is a feature of life and living. Ludwig Wittgenstein, a contemporary Western philosopher, does not think so. He says:

Death is not an event in life: we do not live to experience death. If we take eternity to mean not infinite temporal duration but timelessness, then eternal life belongs to those who live in the present. Our life has no end in just the way in which our visual field has no limits. The temporal immortality of the human soul, that is to say, its eternal survival after death, is not only in no way guaranteed, but this assumption in the first place will not do for us what we always tried to make it do. Is a riddle solved by the fact that I survive forever? Is this eternal life not as enigmatic as our present one?

Poets, philosophers and scientists have remarkably the same approach to portraying death—speculation and imagination, which at times run riot. How else can one chart an uncharted domain that one can never see or enter when alive? Speculation has no defined limits—it can be wild, imaginative, fanciful, or delusional; it can even be sober and restrained. Even so, the truth is an undiscovered enigma— now and perhaps forever. As the poet Percy Shelley says in his famous poem 'On Death':

Who telleth a tale of unspeaking death?
Who lifteth the veil of what is to come?
Who painteth the shadows that are beneath
the wide-winding caves of the peopled tomb?
Or uniteth the hopes of what shall be
with the fears and the love for that which we see?

The Fear of Death

Generally speaking, there appears to be an existential, almost visceral, fear of death in the human race. It is the uncertainty and the absolute 'unknowableness' of what follows the end of life that makes death terrifying. To many, it must also be the fear of retribution—of being plunged into hell for a life lacking in virtue and punctuated by vice. This terrifying belief is expounded by many religions of the world. The following

lines from the poem 'Aubade' by the poet Philip Larkin capture
the dread, fear and horror of death with fierce intensity:

> Waking at four to soundless dark, I stare.
> In time the curtain-edges will grow light.
> Till then I see what's really always there:
> Unresting death, a whole day nearer now,
> Making all thought impossible but how
> And where and when I shall myself die.
> Arid interrogation: yet the dread
> Of dying, and being dead,
> Flashes afresh to hold and horrify.

Not surprisingly, the fear of death is barely considered or
even contemplated when one is young and vigorous—death
seems so far away belonging to another world. It manifests,
however, as one grows older and older. The mist then slowly
lifts, and death, at first seeming remote, comes nearer, soon
becoming a fearful and feared companion towards the end of
one's life.

Yet, there are many exceptions to what I have stated. In
over fifty years of practice as a physician, I have seen so many
patients—young and old—who have met death with courage
and stoicism, with grace and equanimity, without a trace of
manifest fear. Among other features I shall touch upon later, it
is the empathy, compassion and the doctor–patient bond that
helps to condition a dying patient to accept without undue
fear the inevitability of death. Modern medicine is hopelessly
tied up in the way of complex machines and sophisticated
gadgetry. The physician of today, exposed to the glittering
brilliance and capability of modern medicine, concentrates
on treating organ systems and ignores or relegates to the
background the patient as a whole. I see him stay away from
a deathbed, impatient to get on to the next bed where he feels
he could be of better use. After all, what can the doctor do

when death sits at the bedside waiting to take over? I rarely see a doctor holding the hand of a dying patient, sitting by his side, talking to him, consoling him, listening to him, and fortifying him or her gently for what lies ahead. The art and science involving the care of the dying is unfortunately not taught and is learnt and practised by just a few, yet it is one of the core purposes of medicine.

Medicine, Dying and Death

Over a hundred years ago, life on earth was short compared to what it is today. The advances in medicine, both therapeutic and preventive, have played an important role in the present longevity of humans. There is no denying this fact. Modern medicine with its phenomenal advances and with the help of science and technology would aim at humans living even longer and longer. In all Western countries and in many industrialized cities of the East, medicine has declared a war against death. Death has to be fought, with might and main, to the nth degree; it has to be kept at bay, defeated as long as possible. Modern medicine has the wherewithal to do this. There should be no pain, no suffering—they should both be abolished. Society has been conditioned not only to accept this view, but expects it to be realized. It loses sight of the fact that there are limits to medicine. Ivan Illich considers this attitude of medicine to be responsible for cultural iatrogenesis ('*iatros*', in Greek, means 'the physician', genesis means 'to make').

Medicine knows, but must be reminded that death is the only certainty in life, and the hallmark of a good physician is to know when to fight death and when to give in to it. Suffering, in whatever form it takes, is a realistic human response. Like joy and pleasure, pain and suffering are a part of life and living. Unquestionably, pain and suffering need to be alleviated, and medicine has the means to do so. Medical enterprise has, however, declared a war against suffering, wishing to abolish and obliterate it. Patients believe that modern medicine has the power to accomplish this. This has undermined the ability of individuals to face their reality, to express their own values, and to accept the inevitability of pain, impairment, decline and death.

The Vedas and Upanishads teach that each one of us has his or her own cross to bear with regard to pain and suffering, which constitute an integral part of life. According to karma and karmic law, one's actions in the previous life condition the degree of pain and suffering in the present. It is a philosophy that enables people in the East to face suffering and death with less fear and greater equanimity than those in the West. The ability to face death and rob it of its sting is governed to an extent by the religious, philosophical and sociocultural traditions of a particular society or country.

The cultural iatrogenesis that I have mentioned is typically witnessed in critical care units all over the world. Patients who are terminally ill are kept alive on various support systems. This merely prolongs the act of dying and makes death excessively lonely, gruesome, dehumanized, perhaps even obscene and ruinous to the patient and the family. Yet it is very important not to have a cavalier attitude in concluding that an illness in a patient is truly terminal. Occasionally, physicians dub an illness in a patient as terminal, only to have the patient, in due course of time, walk out of the intensive care unit alive and well.

Fortunately, the futility and even the moral wrong of fighting death when death is near and inevitable has been increasingly realized. In almost all units in the world, in a terminal illness, when death approaches, support systems are not instituted or if already instituted are withdrawn. In India, this may not be easy to accomplish. The patient may be too ill to express a coherent wish as to what he or she desires, and the cultural iatrogenesis imbibed by the relatives makes them insist that support systems should be started or not discontinued in spite of repeated explanations as to their futility. The stress of treating very ill patients and also contending with social issues that arise in such situations indeed takes a physical and mental toll on all caring physicians.

Future Medicine and Longevity

Medical research, today, is geared to increase life expectancy and delay and even halt the ageing process. Who knows a hundred years from now, or even earlier, man might mange to live 120–150 years. The world's population would increase first by arithmetic and then by geometric progression— an unmitigated disaster. The Malthusian prophecy would then surely be fulfilled. The resources of the earth would be exhausted, food would be scarce, and famine would stalk the earth. The poor would become poorer, the rich richer; the powerful would feed upon the weak—the ine-quities of the present world would be multiplied several times over.

   Whatever the advances in medicine, death would certainly triumph. A marked increase in the world population and the propensity for extended life would almost certainly encourage a hedonistic existence. More people would strive for power and wealth; more countries would be expansionist. There would be more wars, more pain and suffering. Unprecedented problems would afflict such a future world. Wise men would agree with the poet Lucan when he writes:

> We're all deluded, vainly searching ways
> To make us happy by the length of days;
> For cunningly to make's protract this breath,
> The Gods conceal the happiness of Death.

Discussing Death with the Dying Patient

Should doctors discuss death with patients? It all depends on the patient. There are some patients who wish to discuss death when they realize that the end is near. The physician does this with empathy, skill and reassurance that all discomfort can be countered to a significant extent by palliative care. I remember a young woman dying of advanced ovarian cancer. She wanted to discuss her impending demise, dying and death in general. On my rounds, I would sit by her daily, hold her hand, and we would converse. The conversation often turned philosophical, particularly with what to expect in the afterlife. I painted a picture of a glowing afterlife, not only because I felt it imperative to do so but also because I believe it to be so. One day, just before actually dying, she told me, 'Doctor, my daily conversations with you relieved my discomfort far more than the pain killers the nurses have been giving me'. It was hard to fight back my tears. I managed to do so. After all, an Oslerian equanimity, in spite of the storm of emotions that raged within me, was a dire necessity to reinforce the great fortitude of this dear, dying lady. I realized once again, as I had realized many times before, the importance of the mind–body complex and that the practice of medicine is both an art and a science in equal measure. The continuing ward round was a discussion on these issues; it helped me to blunt to a slight extent the tragedy I had witnessed.

Yet not all patients who are dying, close to death, or suffering from disease where death is inevitable in a few weeks or months wish to discuss death. In the late fifties, when training in the West, I witnessed 'death conferences' when the patient (who was expected to die) and close relatives met the physicians to discuss various aspects relating to the anticipated death of the patient. I tried to follow this when I returned to India by discussing truthfully the serious prognosis in patients who were likely to die. To my surprise, most patients told me specifically that they did not wish to discuss this topic. Others made their wishes clear by interrupting me and changing the conversation. In every case, every aspect of an impending fatal or probably fatal illness needs to be discussed with clarity and truth with the relatives of such patients. But should the physician discuss death with a patient who does not wish to discuss the subject? Very often the patient knows that the end is near but feels and hope that perhaps he or she may be the exception who lives or that he or she would survive longer than what the physician thinks. If that be the patient's wish, who is a physician to destroy that very faint glimmer of hope that helps a patient to bear his or her lot with some degree of fortitude?

The outlook is almost certainly different in the West, where patients are told the absolute truth because they desire to know it and because it is the expected professional attitude. This holds not just for patients who are likely to die very soon but also for those whose life expectancy extends to some months. Even then, the truth need not be divulged brutally (as I have occasionally seen it being done) but can be divulged gently, with the proviso that medicine and surgery can help such patients to live their remaining lives in reasonable comfort, and as best as possible right up to the end.

The Hour of Death

As a physician, I have noted quite a few near-death experiences of patients who survived to relate their experiences. The commonest near-death experience recounted by patients who have survived a cardiac arrest is that of travelling at speed through a very dark tunnel and then seeing a light at the very end of the tunnel. The light is first just a point, but it enlarges so they are ultimately totally enveloped within it. I have heard it described as a blinding light of great beauty.

One patient, I remember, mentioned that during his passage through the tunnel he witnessed a review of his whole life and life incidents. This experience may last just a few minutes in real time but is described as elaborative, rich and uplifting.

The next most common experience recounted is the 'out-of-body experience'. Mr D was an extraordinarily intelligent patient (a linguist who could speak well over a dozen languages). Following repeated surgeries on his abdomen for a bleeding gastric ulcer, Mr D became critically ill. He developed ventricular tachycardia, followed by short bursts of ventricular fibrillation. This was in an era when electrical cardioversion (which restores the normal heart rhythm) was not yet invented. The cause of this complication was a very low potassium level in his blood. He recovered following the prompt administration of potassium. During the time when he very nearly died, he felt that one Mr D was lying on the bed and another Mr D was floating around close to the upper region of a large window. He noticed that after a time his 'double' began to approach him and ultimately merged with his body lying in bed. It was then that he realized that he had recovered. This was my first encounter with an out-of-body experience, and I have had a few similar experiences reported to me by critically ill patients who were near death and who fortunately recovered. Some experience an inner feeling of tranquillity and peace, devoid of bodily sensation, insensate, without fear or pain, and surrounded by unconditional love. There was one individual who saw a world of supernatural beauty, beautiful landscapes filled with heavenly music. He felt reluctant to return to the world from which he seemed to have escaped.

There comes to my mind one patient who reported that he was running at fascinating speed over a beautiful meadow towards his dead grandmother to whom he had been very attached, and who was standing immobile in the far distance. When he came close, the grandmother put her hand out as if asking him to stop—as if to say not now, later. He stopped dead in his track and found himself going back at lightning speed to return to the world.

Does the mind always relate to the body when a person is believed to be dying? Not necessarily so. At times, a patient appears to be dying, and seems to be physically suffering great agony and torment. On recovery, he may relate that he did not feel any agony, distress, or pain, only a pleasant floating sensation of peace and tranquillity.

Sarah Bakewell's biography of Michel Eyquem de Montaigne (who lived in the sixteenth century in France), *How to Live: Or a Life of Montaigne in One Question and Twenty Attempts at an Answer* (2010), illustrates this remarkably well. Montaigne, Bakewell tells us, was thirty-six years old when he was thrown from his horse after another rider collided with him from behind at great speed. He suffered serious injuries to the head and chest and had to be carried home from a considerable distance away. When he recovered consciousness, he seemed to be in significant distress, struggling to breathe, plucking at his clothes, and vomiting large amounts of blood. He was not expected to survive, but he did. In retrospect, he made a remarkable and surprising discovery. Bakewell writes, 'he could enjoy ... delightful floating sensations even while his body seemed to be convulsed, thrashing around in what looked to others like torment'. Montaigne's testimony suggests that there could occur a disconnect between the mind and the body in near-death situations and that those who appear physically distressed may in fact be experiencing delightful floating sensations.

After he had recovered, Montaigne wrote, 'If you don't know how to die, don't worry; Nature will tell you what to do on the spot, fully and adequately. She will do this job perfectly for you; don't bother your head about it'. And it seemed that Montaigne never worried about death again!

Those who have lived through near-death experiences, as also laypeople who have read or heard of them, frequently believe that these experiences give a glimpse of a world beyond and other than our present world. However, most neuroscientists do not think so. They believe that these experiences are related to altered function in a dying or soon-to-die brain. David Hovda, Director, UCLA Brain Injury Research Centre, explains that as the brain begins to change and die, different parts become excited, and one of the parts that becomes excited is the visual system. The description of 'seeing a bright light at the end of the tunnel' is a result of this stimulation. Hallucinations, a dream-like state, the déjà vu phenomenon, as also disturbances in space and time are not uncommon features in pathologies involving the temporal and parietal lobes. Disturbances in function of these areas of the dying brain may well explain the near-death experiences reported by patients.

Jimo Borjigin, a neuroscientist at the University of Michigan, in an article titled 'What It Feels Like to Die' noted that just before the animals died, there was a sudden surge of neurochemicals in the brain; she observed the neurons were secreting new chemicals in large quantities. She is of the opinion this could be the explanation for patients suffering cardiac arrest who describe experiences as 'realer than real'.

Death in the very old who have no clinical evidence of any organic disease is invariably gentle and sweet. They often sleep more and more in the day and all through the night. The sense of hunger and thirst are lost, speech is often lost, and vision is diminished. Touch and hearing are generally the last to go. The patient can no longer be aroused. The clinician and the relative may term this a coma or an unconscious state. Modern researchers in the field believe that it may well be a 'dream state'. In the previously mentioned *Atlantic* article, James Hallenbeck, a palliative-care specialist, describes the end beautifully: 'It's like a storm coming in. The waves started coming up. But you can never say, well, when did the waves start coming up? ...The waves get higher and higher, and eventually, they carry the person out to sea.'

What is the science behind the death of the very aged who on clinical examination show no sign of disease? Each cell in our body has an inbuilt clock within it that determines the time it will function, even in the absence of disease. When the time is up, its lifespan over, the 'bell rings', and the cell dies. This phenomenon is termed apoptosis. With increasing age, an increasing number of cells suffer apoptosis in all organ systems of the body. Perhaps when this cell-death exceeds a certain number, life cannot be sustained and death supervenes.

In spite of all that has been said and written, the actual physical experience of dying remains a mystery. Blaise Pascal has rightly said, '*On mourra seul*' (one dies alone). One cannot even approach the mystery of death without solving the mystery of dying, and medicine, try as it may, is far from doing so.

After Death

Some religions believe in reincarnation—notably the Buddhist and Hindu religions. Both believe in the concept of 'karma'. Let me define karma in simple terms. It is the belief that one reaps in the present life what one has sown in previous lives and that one will reap in a future existence what one sows in the present. How else can one explain the inequities of life, the suffering of the innocent, dreadful diseases afflicting the very young or the virtuous, or calamities befalling people for no apparent reason? Karma says it is the shadow of one's past life that determines what happens in the present.

The Buddhist religion in addition to believing in karma believes in 'bardo'. Bardo is a Tibetan word that simply means a transition or gap between the completion of one situation and onset of another. 'Bar' means 'in between' and 'do' means 'suspended' or 'thrown'.

The word bardo was introduced to the world following the publication and popularity of Sogyal Rinpoche's *The Tibetan Book of Living and Dying* (1994).

Tibetan Buddhists consider existence to be dived into four bardos: the natural bardo of life, the painful bardo of dying, the luminous bardo of *dharmata* (the essence of things as they are), and the karmic bardo of becoming. The luminous bardo of dharmata encompasses the after-death experience of the radiance of the nature of the mind, the luminosity or 'clear light', which manifests as sound, colour and light. The karmic bardo of becoming is the intermediate state lasting right up to the moment one takes on a new birth. It is the transitional zone, the period between death and reincarnation (rebirth).

The Hindu religion is imbued with great philosophy. Its outlook on death, after-death and rebirth is beautifully embodied in the *Katha Upanishad*. In this Upanishad, a young man, Nachiketa, seeks enlightenment on the mystery of death and after-death from Yama, the King of Death. The discourse that ensues between Yama and Nachiketa enlightens this issue. In essence, Yama teaches Nachiketa that death, when it occurs, is of the body but the essence within Man is the *Self,* which is indestructible. It is birthless, deathless, timeless and changeless, even if the body within which it resides is dead. The man who realizes the self within him achieves immortality. He is freed from the otherwise continuous cycle of life and death.

I must quote some passages from this beautiful Upanishad to illustrate what is written above.

> The all-knowing Self was never born,
> Nor will it die. Beyond causes and effect,
> This Self is eternal and immutable.
> When the body dies, the Self does not die.
> If the slayer believes that he can kill

Or the slain believes he can be killed
Neither knows the truth. The eternal Self
Slays not, nor is slain.

Also, listen to what I quote below.

The supreme Self is beyond name and form,
Beyond the senses, inexhaustible,
Without beginning, without end,
Beyond time, space, and causality, eternal,
Immutable. Those who realize the Self
Are forever free from the jaws of death.

And finally, Yama, the King of Death, instructs his pupil
Nachiketa thus:

Now, O Nachiketa, I will tell you
Of this unseen, eternal Brahman, and
What befalls the Self after death. Of those
Unaware of the Self, some are born as
Embodied creatures while others remain
In a lower stage of evolution,
As determined by their own need for growth.

The *Katha Upanishad* teaches that if one realizes the
self, the consciousness within, then 'there is nothing else
to be known', and 'all the knots that strangle the heart are
loosened'. Death comes only to that part of us which was
born into a separate but ephemeral existence. The true real
self within is immortal.

Let me indulge in the utopian thought, in the deep universal
longing, that the human race in the many, many years to come
realizes the *Self*. Then, as John Donne aptly writes:

One short sleep past, we wake eternally
And death shall be no more; Death, thou shalt die.

I feel impelled to end this essay on a personal note. As one who has spent the greater part of his life among the dying and the dead, caring for seriously ill patients in a busy critical care unit, what happens after death continues to be a matter of deep concern. I can temporarily rid myself of this concern when I take a holiday, listen to great music, play the violin, or read a good book. But alas! The concern comes forth again. I have formulated to myself a view, which again will remain a speculation as all other views indeed are.

I feel that after death the 'shell', that is to say the body, whichever way it is disposed of serves to replenish, fertilize and renew the earth. The 'spirit', the self within, goes forth and merges with the 'universal spirit', the force that created and that orchestrates the universe. This universal spirit or force is an indivisible unit, so that one will never be able to identify and meet kindred souls one loved so deeply and so passionately in the world that one has left. I have not realized my true self—not in the way the Upanishads teach. I am, therefore, not fit for immortality. Believing in reincarnation, I shall be reborn into the world (hopefully) in human form— could I or would I have the same parents, the same wife whom I adored and loved above all else in my life on earth? Would I be blessed with the same son and daughter who shared our love, joy and happiness on earth? If I were to be reborn, I would crave that this indeed did happen. And even if it did, we would almost certainly have different physical attributes, and how would we recognize one another or relate to our past existence? This very deep craving and wish, of course, denotes great physical attachments and is a disqualification for immortality!

But then, I do not thirst for immortality. I do not mind at all being reborn in the world. The world is indeed a beautiful place in spite of war, pestilence and famine that ravage parts of it. I love to view a glorious sunrise, a beautiful tropical sunset, the moon on a full moon night glistening on the sea, snow-capped mountains, flowing rivers and the emerald green of lakes hidden within high hills. I am passionate about great music, history, art and books. I love the sound of laughter. I love all the good things of life, but I am not really irrevocably attached to any of them. I could well do without them, but how does one loosen the emotional attachment to people one deeply loves?

Though well past eighty years, physically and mentally reasonably fit, and still at work, I find myself knocking at death's door. I pray that I enter through the door gracefully, purposefully, when it opens. It is amazing how one feels the nearness of the end as one grows older and older. As I mentioned earlier, when young and vigorous, the end seems invisible and enveloped in a haze; when past a certain age, the end is palpably close.

I feel it is important to condition, train and prepare oneself well in advance for death. It is very like preparing for a difficult examination or practising for 'the mile' in an athletic meet. Conditioning oneself brings acceptance to the fact that death is merely an inseparable part of life and living.

Dylan Thomas in his poem 'Do Not Go Gentle into that Good Night' writes:

> Do not go gentle into that good night,
> Old age should burn and rave at close of day;
> Rage, rage against the dying of the light.

Good poetry, but I strongly dispute its content. I would say:

> Go gently into the dark, dark night,
> Close your eyes, smile, and whisper a prayer
> At the passing of the light.

So when the end is nigh, I would wish with Walt Whitman that—

At the last, tenderly,
From the walls of the powerful fortressed house,
From the clasp of the knitted locks, from the keep of the well-
closed doors,
Let me be wafted.

Let me glide noiselessly forth;
With the key of softness unlock the locks—with a whisper,
Set ope the doors O soul.
Tenderly—be not impatient
(Strong is your hold O mortal flesh,
Strong is your hold O love.)

About the Author

Dr Farokh Erach Udwadia is a distinguished physician of international acclaim in the field of Respiratory and Critical Care Medicine. He is at present Emeritus Professor of Medicine at Grant Medical College and JJ Hospital, Bombay; Senior Consultant Physician and Physician in charge of the Intensive Care Unit at the Breach Candy Hospital as also Senior Consultant Physician at the Parsee General Hospital, Bombay.

Besides over 55 contributions to national and international journals, Dr Udwadia has written several major monographs including on *Emergency Medicine, Respiratory Failure, Pulmonary Eosinophilia, Tetanus* and *Principles of Critical Care*. The latter work is the first book of its kind in India and among the very few published in South-East Asia. It is the standard text and reference for critical care all over the country and is now in its third edition. Another monumental monograph titled *Man and Medicine: A History* traces and relates the history of medicine in relation to the history of civilization. It is the only book of its kind in this part of the world. Another important compendium, *Principles of Respiratory Medicine* (2010) is a landmark book in our country.

In 1987 the President of India conferred the Padma Bhushan award on Dr Udwadia for his contribution to medicine. In 1996 he was awarded the Dhanvantri award, the Dr. B.C. Roy National Award for the year 2000 in the category of 'Eminent Medical Teacher', 'The Third Claris International Critical Care Achievement Award – 2005' by Critical Care Education Foundation during the 4th Indo-Australian Training Program in Critical Care Medicine held at Kolkata, December 2005 and 'The Citizen of Mumbai' award by Rotary Club of Bombay, 2008.

He is an astute active physician and remarkably enough, his expert opinion on complicated medical cases is sought after by both, patients and other medical practitioners in our city and country.